"Andy's book will provide hope for those who so desperately need it. These stories of strength and determination are inspiration to keep fighting in our own lives."

— **CÉLINE DION**

Winner of twelve World Music Awards, five Grammy Awards,
seven Billboard Music Awards, and seven American Music Awards

"This book is equally important for anyone with CF, for anyone who has a family member or loved one with CF, or for anyone who loves reading about people with unrelenting spirits and drives to live life to the fullest. I have been involved with the CF Foundation for over twenty years, and the resiliency of each person I have met who is battling this disease amazes and humbles me. A truly great read."

— **CHIPPER JONES**

Eight-time All-Star, 1995 World Series champion, 1999 National League Most Valuable Player,
and first ballot Major League Baseball Hall of Famer in 2018

"I have been lucky enough to have been involved in the community of those stricken by cystic fibrosis and those who search for its cure. It's as deeply rewarding as any experience in my life, and the stories in this lovely book will give you a sense of why. These are tales of warriors who have beaten the odds by making their dreams come true. These are stories that will give you hope. And by buying this book, you will bring us closer to a cure. That is my dream."

— **LEWIS BLACK**

New York Times–*bestselling author, playwright,*
film and voiceover actor, and award-winning comedian

"I became involved with the Cystic Fibrosis Foundation in 2001. I've had the honor to know those afflicted with CF and their families, and the courage I've witnessed with every one of them is nothing short of awe-inspiring. Andy's book is a wonderful testament to that courage."

— **RICHARD MARX**

Grammy Award–winning musician with the distinction of
having a song he wrote or cowrote top the charts in four different decades

"*The CF Warrior Project* will provide hope to those who so desperately need it. These stories are so inspiring."

— GABBY REECE

Former professional volleyball player, TV personality, New York Times–bestselling author, and model

"Being the first *American Ninja Warrior* champion, I'm blown away and deeply inspired by all of the CF warriors' stories of success and their impossible fight to live. This is the epitome of being a true warrior."

— ISAAC CALDIERO

Winner of the seventh season of American Ninja Warrior, *one of the first two Americans to complete all four stages of the National Finals course on the show*

"After spending time with cystic fibrosis warriors throughout the country, I've quickly realized they are the toughest and most resilient people I have ever met. The outlook CF warriors have on life is one that everyone should strive to have."

— COLTON UNDERWOOD

The Bachelor on Season 23 of ABC's The Bachelor *and founder of the Colton Underwood Legacy Foundation*

"The biggest thing that I took away from reading these stories is that every single one of these people with cystic fibrosis chose to rise above their disease and fight back. Their dedication and determination should spark a fire in your life and encourage you to achieve everything you can, and to be thankful for the small victories. It's an amazing compilation of stories about overcoming life's obstacles."

— TENILLE ARTS

2018's "Artist to Watch" by CMT, number-one single on Radio Disney's Country chart in early January 2019, featured on The Bachelor, Rolling Stone, Billboard, Hollywood Life, People *magazine, and beyond*

"Science is beginning to discover what ancient cultures and esoteric teachers have known for thousands of years: the state of your (mind) consciousness is in direct relation to your health and well-being. These are the stories of CF warriors who refused to succumb to a distressful prognosis, and instead thrived through the power of belief."

— MEGAN FOX

Model and actress with roles in more than thirty films,
including the blockbuster hit Transformers

"Stories like the ones published in this book have helped raise money to fund research and educate Congress, and even help a parent raise their child who is struggling with cystic fibrosis. As the old saying goes, sharing is caring. When you care about the entire CF population, as Andy does, you can be certain you'll benefit from his wisdom, his honesty, and his ability to connect your heart to others."

— MARGARETE CASSALINA

Award-winning author of See You at Sunset *and* Beyond Breathing,
motivational speaker, longtime national CF advocate, and CF mother to Jena and Eric

"In this book, you will read stories about the challenges about living with CF and how these resilient individuals have met those challenges. Descriptions of coughing, digestive problems, hospitalizations, questions from peers, and of course, worries about mortality are balanced by accounts of athletic and creative successes, big dreams, and strong family support. Rather than be consumed by the negative, you will read how people with CF have educated and supported the CF community and advocated for others with CF. This is the full picture of life with CF—the struggles and the triumphs. I hope you enjoy these stories of people who have decided that CF stands for 'can't fail.'"

— DRUCY BOROWITZ, MD

Emeritus Professor of Clinical Pediatrics
Jacobs School of Medicine and Biomedical Sciences
University at Buffalo

THE
CF
WARRIOR PROJECT

THE
CF
WARRIOR PROJECT

65

Stories of Triumph
against Cystic Fibrosis

Andy C. Lipman

BOOKLOGIX®

Alpharetta, GA

ISBN: 978-1-61005-955-8 - Paperback
eISBN: 978-1-61005-956-5 - ePub
eISBN: 978-1-61005-957-2 - mobi

Library of Congress Control Number: 2019904138

Printed in the United States of America   0 4 1 8 1 9

♾This paper meets the requirements of ANSI/NISO Z39.48-1992 (Permanence of Paper)

Kalydeco®, Orkambi®, and Symdeko® are registered trademarks of Vertex Pharmaceuticals Incorporated; Pulmozyme® is a registered trademark of Genentech, Inc.; Mucomist® is a registered trademark of Beximco Pharmaceuticals Ltd.; TOBI® is a registered trademark of Novartis Pharmaceuticals Corp.; Top Model® is a registered trademark of Pottle Productions, Inc.; Bactrim® is a registered trademark of Sun Pharmaceutical Industries; Love To Breathe® is a registered trademark of Somer Love; ThAIRapy™ is a registered trademark of Hill-Rom Services PTE Ltd.; Make-A-Wish® is a registered trademark of the Make-A-Wish Foundation of America; WebMD® is a registered trademark of WebMD, Inc.; Emmy Award® is a registered trademark of the National Academy of Television Arts & Sciences and The Academy of Television Arts & Sciences.

Photo of Claire Wineland courtesy of POPSUGAR Beauty; photo of Jake Baker courtesy of Pam Baker; photo of Kayden Stephenson courtesy of complikayden; photo of Teena Mobley courtesy of Cinnematic X; photo of Harry Coffey courtesy of Darren Weir Racing - Horse Signoff; photo of Angela DeStasio courtesy of Dominick Spolitino; photo of Michael Rowe courtesy of Josh Borgmann; photo of Ben Mudge courtesy of Martin Irvine Photography; photo of Bianca Nicholas courtesy of Emma Samms; photo of Andy Simmons courtesy of James Musselwhite; photo of Beth Sufian courtesy of James Passamano; photo of Travis Flores courtesy of Clement Souyri; photo of Jerry Cahill courtesy of Brand 7, LLC: Chase Cabral; photo of Elizabeth "Libby" Hankins courtesy of Alisa Lynn; photo of Alex Pangman courtesy of Lisa MacIntosh.

For my wife, Andrea, who encouraged me
to take on this project and to never look back. I love you.

CONTENTS

THE 65 ROSES STORY

Choosing sixty-five warriors from the more than five hundred we interviewed for this book was extremely difficult; however, making the decision to go with that exact number was a relatively easy one. While in most worlds the number sixty-five is pretty insignificant, in the cystic fibrosis community, it's as iconic as Jackie Robinson's number forty-two to an avid baseball fanatic.

The story of how sixty-five became a symbol of the cystic fibrosis community all began coincidentally enough in 1965, when Mary G. Weiss, who was living in Canada with her husband and two sons, finally received a diagnosis of cystic fibrosis for her youngest son, Richard (Ricky), who had been struggling his first four years with frailness. Soon after, his older brother, Arthur, was also diagnosed with the disease. To make matters worse, Mary did not realize that she was pregnant at the time with Anthony, who would eventually be diagnosed with CF, too.

Mary was told by the doctor that the prognosis was bleak. She was advised to take the two boys home, love on them, and do not expect them to live more than seven years. Mary ignored the advice, though, and would not give up. She soon moved the boys to Florida, hoping the warmer weather would help them. She became a volunteer for the Cystic Fibrosis Foundation, and was soon responsible for calling multiple organizations to seek financial support for CF research. A year later, she founded the Palm Beach Chapter of the Cystic Fibrosis Foundation, the first chapter in the state of Florida. However, it's what happened one day in 1965 that has an even bigger significance.

Ricky, who was four at the time, listened closely as she made each call. After several calls, he walked into the room and told his mom, "I know what you are working for." Mary was in a bit of shock, because her little boy did not know what she was doing, nor did he even know that he had cystic fibrosis.

With some apprehension, Mary asked, "What am I working for, Ricky?"

His response became one of CF folklore: "You are working for sixty-five roses."

Mary was speechless as tears began running down her cheeks. "Yes, Ricky," she stammered. "I'm working for sixty-five roses."

Ricky would succumb to the disease in 2014 at the age of fifty-two, while his older brother, Arthur, would lose the fight to CF in 1996 at the age of thirty-six. Anthony, the youngest of the three and now in his fifties, continues to live with the disease. Mary passed away in April of 2016, but not before she and Ricky would coin a phrase that would live on long after them.

Since that moment in 1965, the phrase "sixty-five roses" has been used by children of all ages, and has caught on in places as far away as Australia, to describe the disease that is just as difficult to live with as it is to pronounce.

Cystic fibrosis affects anywhere from seventy thousand to eighty thousand people around the world. While breakthrough drugs have been discovered and approved over recent years, we still do not have a cure.

This book is dedicated to Mary, her family, and all of the CF warriors, past and present, who never gave up hope in the fight against "sixty-five roses."

FOREWORD

By reading the introduction to Andy's book, you are now familiar with the origin of the "sixty-five roses" story in which Ricky, a four-year-old boy, told his mother, Mary, that he knew she was working for sixty-five roses because he could not pronounce the disease that he would spend a lifetime fighting. My brother's story inspired thousands of people around the world to raise millions of dollars to benefit those with cystic fibrosis.

My name is Anthony Weiss, and, at age fifty-three, I am the youngest of the three Weiss brothers, and Mary was my mother. My two brothers and I were born with cystic fibrosis during a time when the average life expectancy was only seven years of age. Knowing the statistics, the doctors told my mom to take us home and love on us, for we had no future. Despite these dire predictions, we each graduated college, married, and had successful business careers as commodity traders. Sadly, I am now the only surviving brother of the Weiss family.

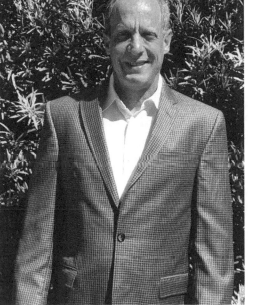

Anthony Weiss

My mom was instrumental in the creation of the "sixty-five roses" moniker and conservatively raised over $10–$15 million during her lifetime. Her ongoing campaign for public awareness and better treatments inspired a generation of CF families. Her dream was to find a cure, and we get one step closer each day to realizing her goal.

One question that I am often asked: "How did my brothers and I survive for so long against insurmountable odds?" There is no doubt that genetics and medical advances played a significant role, but I believe that attitude is often an underappreciated critical component to surviving cystic fibrosis. Mom, in fact, instilled in each of us the will to not only survive this disease, but to thrive despite it. We were not allowed to use CF as a crutch, and were encouraged from day one to aspire to live as normal a life as possible. I am proud to say that my brothers and I never allowed this horrible disease, nor the immensely negative data that went along with it, to define who we were.

An example of this is when I started my first full-time job after college. While completing paperwork, the benefits manager asked if I wanted to invest in the 401(k) plan for retirement, which for the average person is probably a no-brainer. The chances of me living to age sixty-five—the number that has followed my family for years—were nonexistent, and candidly, I would much rather have used that disposable income on dating women and drinking alcohol, as those were higher priorities at the time. But, against the prevailing realities, I opted into the company's retirement plan, which reflected my unyieldingly positive approach to living in the face of adversity and overwhelmingly negative statistics. My action was no different than the lifetime of choices that I've made, such as doing my daily therapy, taking my medications, and proactively treating infections.

Andy's book and the sixty-five warriors featured in it are testaments to the importance of believing in oneself and opening up our minds to explore what is possible. I hope you enjoy this journey together as we inspire others to keep on fighting, and know that we are only limited by our own expectations.

—*Anthony Weiss*

PREFACE

When I was six years old, I got the itch for athletic competition. But no sooner did I get off the running blocks than I was stopped by coughing fits. Nothing was more frustrating than watching my classmates run ten to twelve laps around the school gymnasium when I could not even complete one. While most of my peers looked forward to hitting the gym in the middle of the day, I absolutely dreaded it.

It was embarrassing having my mom write notes excusing me from participating in PE because of my CF. Both my parents and my medical team were concerned about me becoming out of breath and struggling to keep up with the other kids my age; however, I don't think anyone was as perplexed as me. The questions that I mulled in my head were ones that a grammar school student should never have to ask: "What is wrong with me? What does cystic fibrosis mean to my life? Why do I have to do things that other kids don't, and why can't I do things that other kids can?" I was void of hope that I could succeed in life, much less athletics.

That was, until my faith was restored at the one place where, ironically, my hopes and dreams were often crushed: the doctor's office. I was eight years old and in the midst of receiving more bad news from Dr. Caplan at Grady Hospital in downtown Atlanta, Georgia. I had just done a sputum test because I had been coughing a lot more than normal. After I was forced to bring up some mucus, Dr. Caplan sent me over to the waiting room while he sent the sample down to the lab to determine which bacteria was responsible for further damaging my already compromised young lungs.

I sat there deflated (forgive the pun) as I stared at the sad stacks of back issues of *Newsweek, Time,* and a whole bunch of other grown-up magazines that littered the waiting room table. Then, I looked up, and noticed—no, became *mesmerized* by a poster on the wall. It featured some nameless strongman whom I think was advertising a weight-gain drink, but I had never seen a man with such hulking, defined muscles. He looked like one of the superheroes from my comic books. It was awesome! In my reverie, I began to wonder what he had done to get such chiseled arms and looked down at my own, which resembled thinly cooked spaghetti noodles, due mostly to one of cystic fibrosis's major symptoms, malnutrition.

"He has cystic fibrosis," my mom said, smiling. I looked up at her, confused. "Yep," she said, nodding toward the poster. "*That* guy." My heart welled up with the joy of possibility, of *hope*. I couldn't help but smile embarrassingly wide as I realized I *too* could have chiseled arms and be on a poster! Every dream I had was in play. I did not have a worry in the world. In my mind, I would be just as strong as the guy on the poster someday. I had never heard of working out and just assumed I would eventually just transform into a body double for Arnold Schwarzenegger. It was as if cystic fibrosis was just a phase in my life that would eventually pass, like my love of *Star Wars* action figures.

Unfortunately, that taste of unbridled joy was soon smothered by an encyclopedia article I read later when I was nine. The article informed me that people with cystic fibrosis were only expected to live twenty-five years, and I was devastated. I thought everyone lived into their seventies and eighties; I was only expected to live a third of that. The memory of the muscular man on the poster took a backseat to the harsh reality of living with the deadliest genetic disease in the United States.

As a young boy with cystic fibrosis growing up in the early eighties, my parents constantly encouraged me to stay healthy so I could live a long, quality life while fighting my genetic disease. While their remarks were well-intentioned, I'd never heard of anyone with CF living long enough to attend college, much less feature even a speck of gray hair. I was frustrated because I felt like my parents wanted me to do something that was impossible. My dad, for example, would ask every day if I had ventured outside the house to do something physically active with my friends. My

answer not only felt like a dagger penetrating his heart, but one that permeated mine as well.

I was small, skinny, and coughed so much that I would draw the attention of onlookers. I began to notice differences between me and everyone else, like taking pills and doing postural drainage. I also noticed that no one coughed like I did, and that scared me. I wanted to ask questions, but I was scared to hear the answers. So, I just started answering them myself. Would I go away to college one day? No. Would I have my own family? No. Would I be old enough to run for president one day? No. I even had the notion that the reason that everyone called me Andy instead of my given name, Andrew, was because Andy was a kid's name, and I would not live long enough to reach adulthood. The thought of dying young consumed me. I hated my disease, my parents for giving it to me, and God for not taking it away.

Unbeknownst to me, treatments were sparse in the seventies and eighties, and therefore the median life expectancy for someone with cystic fibrosis when I was born was in the early teens. At an age when a majority of the population was learning how to read and write or ride a bike, someone with this life-shortening disease was already facing a midlife crisis. I also did not realize that my sister, Wendy, born just three years before me, had died after only sixteen days from cystic fibrosis.

My parents never sat me down for a family meeting to discuss my sister. The only hints I was given that I even had a sister were those difficult days in December and January that marked the anniversaries of her birthday and the day she died. Those were the times that my mom would remind me of how fortunate I was to be alive. As a kid, I had difficulty relating the death of my sister to the fact that I should feel lucky to be alive with a terminal disease. There was one chief reason that I could not make the correlation. My parents, along with my many cousins, aunts, and uncles, agreed that it was crucial to my sanity and theirs that I not learn of my sister's cause of death. After all, Wendy and I were the only two members of our family to share this monstrous illness. It was not until I was twenty-five years old that I was finally able to get my mom to reveal the long-kept family secret to me.

Since I never knew my sister, nor that she had the disease until I was much older, I did not know a soul who had cystic fibrosis. It wasn't that CF warriors didn't exist, it's just that they rarely survived past high school. Therefore, their stories were rarely published, especially since the social-media era had yet to emerge. I still joke that the only thing positive back then regarding cystic fibrosis was the "positive" diagnosis of CF provided by the sweat test, the main assessment that determines whether someone has the disease based on the cystic fibrosis transmembrane conductance regulator (CFTR) protein. People with CF laugh. Civilians, not so much.

Cystic fibrosis in the simplest terms is a genetic lung disease that can only be inherited if each parent has the CF gene. Even then, the odds are one in four that the embryo will have the disease. Cystic fibrosis affects more than seventy thousand people worldwide. While many outsiders see CF as only a lung disease, there are many more complications that can arise, including but not limited to pancreatic insufficiency and pancreatitis, sinusitis and nasal polyps, liver disease, osteoporosis and arthritis, male—and in some cases female—infertility, nail clubbing (due to a lack of oxygen in the blood), malnutrition, increased risk for digestive-tract cancers, hemoptysis (coughing up blood), and CF-related diabetes (CFRD). The list of symptoms reads like a WebMD® cocktail.

While the complications present an already difficult list of symptoms, it's nothing compared to the work that a patient has to put in to stay healthy. For those of us with digestive issues, we take thirty to forty pills a day with meals, which mostly consist of digestive enzymes. For those of us with pulmonary issues, our respiratory therapies can range from a mere thirty minutes to a robust two to three hours. Some of us are on IV antibiotics for another several hours a day. Those of us with CF-related diabetes also have to test our insulin several times a day. Then there are nasal therapies to fight sinusitis. Add to that, many of us are required to see our doctors at least quarterly to perform a pulmonary function test, which determines if we need to stay the course or have a "tune-up," a

CF patient's term for spending time in a hospital administering intravenous antibiotics. Given the choice of diseases to have, I think it's fair to say CF would be at or near the bottom for most people.

Like every younger generation before us, adults often asked us what we wanted to do when we grew up. For parents of those with CF, all they wanted was for us to "grow up." I was no different from anyone else when I was a little boy. I had dreams. I wanted to be a veterinarian. My mom laughs that I once exclaimed to my entire family that I wanted to be a "veteran" when I grew up. That all changed when a book gave me my prognosis. It felt as if my dreams were crushed by an eighteen-wheeler. People still asked the question, but my answer changed to "I don't know what I want to do when I grow up," which loosely translated meant "What's the point?"

Adults were not the only ones asking questions. My grammar-school peers asked me some very difficult CF-related questions that oftentimes left me in tears. "Why are you so salty when you sweat?" "Are you contagious?" And my absolute favorite, "Andy, are you going to die?"

I don't think their questions were intended to be cruel. Kids are just very curious, and filters aren't exactly their strong suit. But, on top of that, neither children nor adults were very educated about CF back then. There wasn't an internet to do research on, and encyclopedias weren't very up to date. Young cystic fibrosis patients like me,

whether we liked it or not, were not only tasked with the responsibility of surviving, we had to act as Wikipedia as well.

It wasn't until 1986 that cystic fibrosis finally gained some notoriety when a movie made from a 1983 book with the same name, *Alex: The Life of a Child*, premiered on the ABC television network. The book was about Alex Deford, who was born in the early seventies and passed away in 1980 from cystic fibrosis. Alex was the daughter of the famous national sports columnist and NPR commentator Frank Deford, who himself passed away just recently. Alex died at the age of eight, and like it or not, that became the stereotype for those with the disease at that time.

I struggled for the next decade plus with constant fear of having a disease with an early expiration date. I eventually took advantage of the ThAIRapy™ Vest, a machine that took the place of my parents doing my postural drainage. The device allowed me to go away to college. Not far, mind you. I attended the University of Georgia.

Unfortunately, I was not prepared to introduce the world to my cystic fibrosis. I had kept it mostly quiet growing up. In college, I found that luxury to be impossible as peers saw and heard the loud vest machine that sat in my room. Classmates and fraternity brothers asked why I took pills with meals, and people who tried to look out for me in many cases treated me like a fragile doll rather than a human being. I became depressed, stopped doing my treatments and taking my drugs, and secluded myself in my room for days at a time. I nearly failed out of school.

That is when I had an epiphany. What if the poster I'd witnessed as a youngster was not as farfetched as I had made it seem? I realized that if I put in the work and used my differences to help others, I could change my own prognosis and create a legacy that could change the way people view those with cystic fibrosis. I dislodged the pity handcuffs, found my way to the gym, and persevered inside the classroom and out. I transformed from a scrawny CF victim to a powerful CF warrior.

Fast-forward about twenty years. It was a cold October day. We were finishing another successful charity tournament in memory of my sister. A father and his son came up to my wife, Andrea. I heard the father ask her if this was a charity event for cystic fibrosis. Being that his son, Toby, had CF, I had to keep at least six feet of distance in order to mitigate the possibility of bacterial cross-contamination between cystic fibrosis patients. "Toby," the man said to his boy, "look at Mr. Lipman here. You can be strong, just like him."

Now, my physique paled to that of the man on the poster holding the weight-gain drink, but the look of disbelief on Toby's face as his head darted between his father and me suggested that I, somehow, had become someone else's poster!

I eventually figured out that the man on the poster was most likely a fitness model who was paid to endorse the drink and didn't have cystic fibrosis. In fact, there weren't even clinics to care for adults with CF back then, because there weren't many living that long. Even in my early thirties, I was attending children's clinics full of Disney books, video games, and twenty-piece jigsaw puzzles. When I visited the University of Cincinnati Children's Hospital in Cincinnati, Ohio, I was the only patient asked to have my parking validated, the only patient who asked that something other than *Lady and the Tramp* be played on the waiting-room television, the only one to be asked by the x-ray technician how my child was doing.

But, without exaggeration, my mom's little white lie regarding the man on the poster changed my mindset, transforming the sick child who could not complete a lap in his grammar school gymnasium to a poised forty-five-year-old man who, for two-plus decades, has been competing in ten-kilometer races. And, thanks to medical advances and the internet, we don't need to search hard for literally thousands of amazing stories out there of doctors, nurses, athletes, firemen, policemen, and countless college graduates, all of whom have cystic fibrosis, and many of whom are still killing it in their forties, fifties, sixties, and even seventies!

I interviewed individuals all over the world, from Australia to South America, desperately retrieving as many of these firsthand accounts as I could for two reasons: first, to give parents a little instant hope as they guide their CF warriors through a medical labyrinth fraught with psychological pitfalls, and second, to arm these same parents with highly readable stories of brilliance and inspiration that can be shared aloud with their children as they stare longingly at an elusive poster, contemplating their own potential, which, you will find in the pages that follow—from a young woman who fought for and eventually succeeded in having a breakthrough CF drug approved in her country, to a man who, after several attempts, was able to climb Mount Everest—is seemingly unlimited.

GLOSSARY OF TERMS

Bacterial Cross-Contamination
The possibility of one CF patient passing on a bacteria to another. The Cystic Fibrosis Foundation currently recommends six feet of distance between patients because of this concern.

CF
Acronym for cystic fibrosis.

CFRD
Acronym for cystic fibrosis–related diabetes, a unique type of diabetes that is common amongst people with CF.

Cystic Fibrosis
A lung disease that also affects the digestive system, sinuses, liver, and reproductive system. Cystic fibrosis is the deadliest genetic disease in the United States. In order for a child to have CF, each parent must have the CF gene, and then there is a 25 percent chance the child will have CF, a 50 percent chance the child will be a carrier, and a 25 percent chance the child will neither be a carrier nor a patient.

FEV
Acronym for forced expository volume. Measures how much air a person exhales during a forced breath. With regard to cystic fibrosis, the FEV1, or the amount of air a person is capable of blowing out in the first second, is normally the most important statistic measured when determining one's lung-disease stage.

Hemoptysis
Bleeding from the lungs and another potential symptom of cystic fibrosis.

IVF
Acronym for in-vitro fertilization, a medical procedure done by doctors to attempt to help a family that is having difficulty getting pregnant naturally. Less than 5 percent of male CF patients have the ability to have children without the use of fertility treatments due to the lack of a vas deferens, which is the bridge that moves sperm from the testicles to the urethra. Females can also have a difficult time getting pregnant or carrying a baby full-term due to the effects of cystic fibrosis.

Kalydeco®, Orkambi®, and Symdeko®
Breakthrough CF drugs from Vertex Pharmaceuticals.

Meconium Ileus
A blocked intestine, a common symptom of cystic fibrosis.

Newborn Screening

Public program to screen a newborn to see if he or she has a genetic disease like cystic fibrosis.

PFT

Acronym for pulmonary function test, which is used to gauge someone's lung function with cystic fibrosis.

Postural Drainage

A procedure where the patient gets into certain positions and either self-administers or has someone else administer therapy to loosen the mucus in the patient's lungs. This is often done by cupping one's hands and hitting the patient's sides, back, and front, until the patient is able to cough up the sputum.

Pneumothorax

When air or gas is stuck in the cavity between the lungs and the chest wall, causing the lung to collapse.

Tune-Up

A hospital stay for cystic fibrosis patients that involves IV antibiotics.

TOBI®

Inhaled oral antibiotic.

Vest

A device used by many CF patients, often two or three times a day between thirty to forty-five minutes each time, that helps loosen the phlegm in one's lungs.

DISCLAIMER

Please discuss with the patient's doctor before making any changes to his or her health routine. Everyone's bodies work differently, so what might work for one person may not work for another.

KAYDEN STEPHENSON

Age: 22 **Resides:** Oklahoma, United States **Age at diagnosis:** 15 months

Kayden was on American Idol *Season 12 and used that platform to raise awareness for CF. The Tulsa, Oklahoma, native and alternative R&B singer currently has 185,000 Instagram followers. He recently dropped a mixtape called "Kollection" under his hugely popular social-media account complikayden.*

"I have a lot more baggage and things to do in my daily regimen, so I always have a chip on my shoulder, but I believe that's what helps me thrive."

BRIANNA "BREE" LABIAK

Age: 15

Resides: South Carolina, United States

Age at diagnosis: 21 months

2017 South Carolina Governor's Cup state champion; currently in second place at the Regional East Coast Championships in Explorer Women's Longboard and third in Explorer's Girls for the 2017/2018 NSSA National Championships; finished third in both the Under 16 and Under 18 divisions in Atlantic City at the USA Surfing Prime East in October 2018; considered one of the top-three surfers on the East Coast of the United States in the Under 16 and Under 18 divisions at the age of fifteen; will surf in the World Surf League Junior Pros in 2019

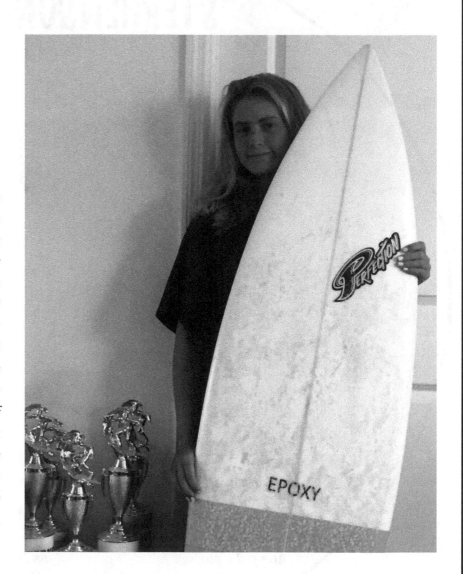

"I never really think twice about having CF and surfing. Beating CF is something I've always wanted to do."

Bree Labiak's journey to surfing stardom began, interestingly enough, in Minooka, Illinois, a small town without a single beach an hour away from Chicago. Bree did not have the typical CF symptoms of failure to thrive or salty skin. In fact, her pediatrician was always reassuring Bree's parents that she was growing just fine. However, her mom, Lynn, said she had a sixth sense that something was wrong, because Bree was defecating quite a bit more than the average infant. Around twenty-one months, her rectum prolapsed from all of the bowel movements, and they realized that she was not properly digesting meals. Soon after, Bree was diagnosed with cystic fibrosis.

Lynn was in absolute shock. She first learned about CF in college when she met a sickly-looking freshman who died a few months into the school year from cystic fibrosis. "That's all I had in my head [when Bree was diagnosed]. I was so mad at God. I was forty and finally blessed with a child." Lynn says she learned to accept the diagnosis over time. Instead of demanding a pity party, she made sure Bree would enjoy what life has to offer. "Bree will not read about adventures in a book—she will experience them herself. Whatever I am able to afford, she will do."

Bree's doctor had faith in his patient as well, telling Lynn that Bree was born at a time when progressive treatments were available, and her health was stable enough to live a long life.

Bree and Lynn faced some family drama in Illinois that weighed heavily on Bree, so Lynn moved the two of them to Conway, South Carolina, where Lynn, a quartermaster, took a job as an evidence technician in the police department. Following the move, Lynn helped her daughter find relief from her anxiety and depression when she purchased the movie *Soul Surfer* for the two to watch.

"Little did I know, that movie would be my inspiration, my driving force to try something new," says Bree. "It was about a girl named Bethany Hamilton. Bethany was thirteen when a shark bit off her left arm. When I saw that Bethany continued to surf even [without] her arm, I realized the tough times I faced in Illinois were nothing compared to what Bethany went through."

Lynn was surprised that Bree took an interest in the sport. The closest beaches were nearly an hour away, and Bree had not even wanted to swim when they moved to Conway, much less surf. In 2011, after seeing how excited Bree was to try surfing, Lynn contacted the Mauli Ola Foundation, a national organization that connects kids with cystic fibrosis to pro surfers as an opportunity to learn to surf and provide hope and improved health. Mauli Ola called Bree and said Nissen Osterneck, a professional MMA fighter and big-wave surfer, was in Myrtle Beach and willing to teach her how to surf.

A few weeks later, Bree met Nissen and surfed with him. "I was up on my surfboard the first wave I ever caught, which is really rare! That moment when I jumped into the ocean, I could tell that surfing was what I was meant to do with my life." Nissen called Bree a "natural" on the board. Not only did Bree enjoy the sport, but her health benefitted too, as saline from the ocean has shown to help people with cystic fibrosis to limit lung infections.

It did not take Bree long to get good at her new craft. Lynn drove her daughter out to Pawley's Island, Surfside Beach, and Myrtle Beach nearly every day for her to spend a few hours practicing. The following year, at the age of nine, Bree surfed in her first amateur competition and got fourth place, which only motivated her to do better. In her next contest, she got third. By 2014, she was winning nearly every competition, and guestimates that she has won more than one hundred amateur surfing competitions.

She is grateful to her grandma Bev (Lynn's mom) as well as Lynn for always being there for her and encouraging her to stay healthy by taking her enzymes and doing her vest. She says that whenever she deals with her CF or anxiety issues, they preach to her to have faith in God and to stay the course. Lynn often tells her, "Live your life. Experience your life, good and bad. You are a kid, and you just happen to have CF."

To date, Bree says her symptoms are under control and her FEV1 is stable at around 85 percent. She credits one thing in particular to feeling so well. "I can definitely tell that surfing clears my lungs. I can breathe better, I can function better, and I feel better."

As far as her feelings about conquering CF while trying to navigate a surfing career, Bree overcomes those concerns like just another big wave. "I never really think twice about having CF and surfing. Beating CF is something I've always wanted to do."

KAYLEIGH MACGREGOR

Age: 22   **Resides:** Wisconsin, United States   **Age at diagnosis:** Birth

Kayleigh, who has raced against and beaten the likes of Olympians Breezy Johnson and Stacy Cook, has made it to both the U16 and U19 Junior Championships twice between the ages of fifteen and nineteen. She was also invited to compete in the US National Championships through the International Ski Federation (FIS) against some of the best skiers in the world, including reigning Olympic Gold Medalist and World Cup Champion Mikaela Shiffrin. Kayleigh, a competitive collegiate skier at the University of Wisconsin–Madison, recently won three United States Collegiate Ski and Snowboard Association (USCSA) races. She currently coaches elite athletes and is a personal trainer for ski-specific athletes.

"Embrace the suffering, don't ignore it.
The more the pain is ignored, the greater it becomes."

GRACE ROSE BAUER

Age: 16

Resides: California, United States

Age at diagnosis: 2 weeks

Designer of the Rosie G clothing line; written up in Forbes Magazine *at age twelve; hosted a small fashion show on the Hallmark Channel as well as the Harry Connick Jr. show; helped raise over $300,000 to help CF research by benefiting her Grace Rose Foundation and the Cystic Fibrosis Foundation; helps host the live auction for the California Winemasters, the largest cystic fibrosis charity event in California, for which she is the CF ambassador*

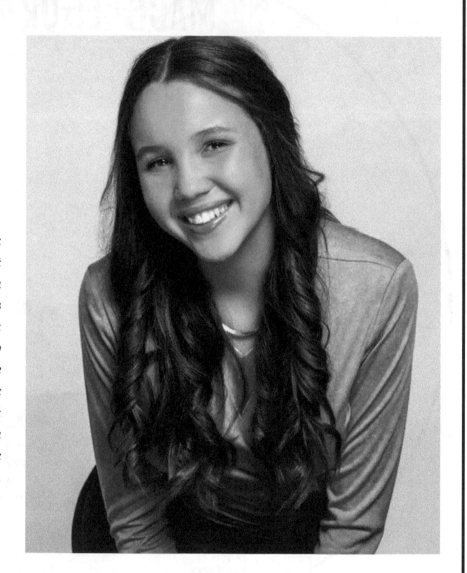

"You might as well deal with it 'in style'!"

Grace Rose Bauer's family has hosted a fashion fundraiser for cystic fibrosis every year since the feisty CF warrior was born. However, it's Grace Rose herself who now does a majority of the hosting. For the tenth annual event, she designed the entire collection. While all the clothes were auctioned off, people wanted to buy more and continue to support her cause. So, she started a website with a small collection and hasn't looked back.

Today, the sixteen-year-old has her own clothing line, Rosie G, which is carried in Nordstrom's and other major department stores. The proceeds from each design she sells go to the Cystic Fibrosis Foundation. Supported by her mom, Leah, a designer herself, Grace Rose's goal is simple: to "#cureCF #instyle."

Born in New Orleans, Louisiana, her family moved to Los Angeles after Hurricane Katrina destroyed a large portion of her hometown. The Rosie G line represents casual comfort and is inspired by her love for the two cities. She wants it to be clothing young girls can wear all the time.

The name "Rosie G" comes from when, as a child, she'd put on lip gloss, get dressed up, and sing and dance in the mirror. "Everyone would say, 'Oh look, here comes Rosie G!'" she says, and proudly admits that she often channels her love of performance when she is doing interviews, speaking at events, or simply encouraging other young girls to pursue their dreams.

The challenge of balancing her career as a designer and public face of CF with her academic responsibilities is made all the more impressive when you consider the regimen of thirty to forty medications she has to follow over the course of the day. And yet, she sort of shrugs it off, saying that her friends, her family, her pug ("Buddy Holly"), and now a clothing line all motivate her to stay the difficult course.

"Everyone has something to deal with," she says. "You might as well deal with it 'in style'!"

MADI VANSTONE

Age: 17

Resides: Toronto, Ontario, Canada

Age at diagnosis: 8 months

Recipient of Cystic Fibrosis Canada Teen Advocacy award; SickKids Hospital ambassador; InvisiYouth global brand ambassador; Global Genes™ International Teen Champion of Hope; advocate in helping get breakthrough drugs funded in Canada

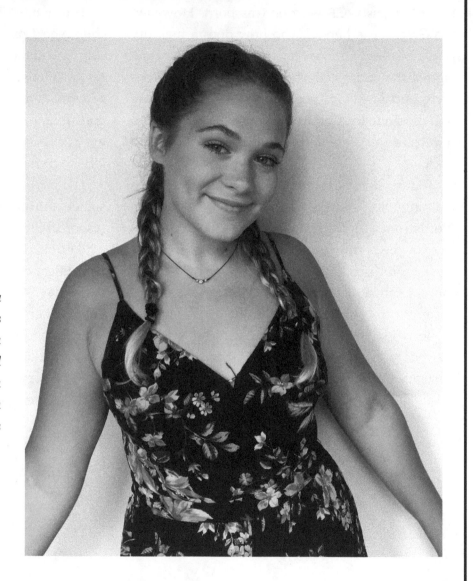

"I'm living my life the way I'm supposed to be, and it sucks that there are people out there with CF who can't have that, too."

When Madi Vanstone was just seventeen months old in 2003, the family's first team—"Madi's Maniacs"—walked at the Toronto Zoo to raise awareness for CF. They have done that every year since, and have raised nearly $50,000 for Cystic Fibrosis Canada. More importantly, Madi and her family's foray into CF activism lit a fire that continues to burn brightly and has established Madi as an important voice for children in Canada battling the disease.

Madi recalls when she knew she was not like everyone else. "I realized not everyone did treatments and took lots of pills like me," she says. "I remember asking my mom why God gave me CF. My mom said because I was brave enough to handle it, and that I had a wonderful sister who would be there by my side and a great mommy and daddy who would help in every way they could." Madi remembers that her conversation with her mom made her believe everything was going to be okay.

Madi has been hospitalized for approximately four to five weeks every year since her diagnosis. At age eleven, Madi agreed to participate in a blind study for the breakthrough drug Kalydeco. Though the study was blind, she could tell by her improving health that she was on the real drug. "I felt great," she says. "My bellyaches subsided along with my headaches, and my energy soared." When the trial ended, it looked as though she would have to come off the drug, as neither her family's insurance nor the province where they were living, Ontario, would help cover it. Most drugs for the disabled are covered under the Ontario Drug Program; however, special, expensive drugs like Kalydeco are normally covered under something called the Exceptional Access Program. Kalydeco was not covered by either program, putting Madi's health in danger.

When the pharmaceutical company, Vertex, discounted the drug, Madi's dad's insurance agreed to pay part, but the family was still responsible for the hefty sum of $7,000 per month to keep her on the drug.

The people of Madi's community sprang into action, organizing galas, park concerts, and raffles. Her mother, Beth, created a video and shared it on Facebook, describing the disease, Madi's struggles, and the new "miracle drug." Soon, complete strangers were sending money to help cover the costs of the drug. During this outpouring of support, a friend of Madi's who was fighting for government approval of a life-saving cancer drug invited Madi's family to join her at Queen's Park, the provincial government, to rally. They did. Madi saw an opportunity for a long-term solution. "I decided to write to our member of Parliament Jim Wilson," she says. "He said he would take it to Queen's Park."

Beth remembers how the community came together at the first rally, which was designed to help their friend get approval for her cancer drug. "The rally was at Queen's Park, which is Ontario's provincial Parliament home. There were a number of media there, as well as the members of provincial Parliament (MPPs) and the premiere of Ontario and health ministers. After the initial trip to Queen's Park to rally and the overwhelming media coverage received, Madi realized that she was being given a platform to make a difference. For whatever reason, the media and the public were interested and passionate about this story. There were phone messages from the media for Madi to discuss her story. She was excited to perhaps be able to make a difference for the others with approved mutations struggling for coverage."

Their fight continued. "My mom and I decided we should rally again. Then, my school got involved, and they all wrote letters and signed petitions to have Kalydeco covered by the province. Then my classmates accompanied me to Queen's Park. I had also shared a letter I had written to the premiere to write for one of Toronto's largest papers. She printed the letter and had me on the front page three separate times."

When Beth and Madi attended the second rally at Queen's Park, their member of Parliament once again raised Madi's story in the House, and she was acknowledged by the premiere during her response.

"I built enough clout to hold my own press conference, and Queen's Park went nuts! It took a lot of pressure, but eventually the drug was covered for me and any others who needed it."

Madi still receives letters of thanks from those people whose health was positively affected by her campaign; however, she is not done. Orkambi, like Kalydeco, is also a breakthrough CF drug that is not provided for people with CF in her community. While Madi does not need this drug, she is aware that it would greatly help other CF patients. Therefore, Madi made her case for them. "I'm living my life the way I'm supposed to be, and it sucks that there are people out there with CF who can't have that, too."

Madi continues to not only speak at fundraisers and events, she has participated in every study she has been asked to do in order to help get the CF community closer to a cure. "I am stronger than I ever would have been had I not had to face the challenges I face every day," she says about how CF has impacted her resolve. "I am compassionate and caring, as I know how it feels to be wishing things could be better. And, I plan to fight the disease within me as hard as I fight for a cure for our community." She continues, "We are stronger than we know, and there is always some fight left. Let the ones who love you help you."

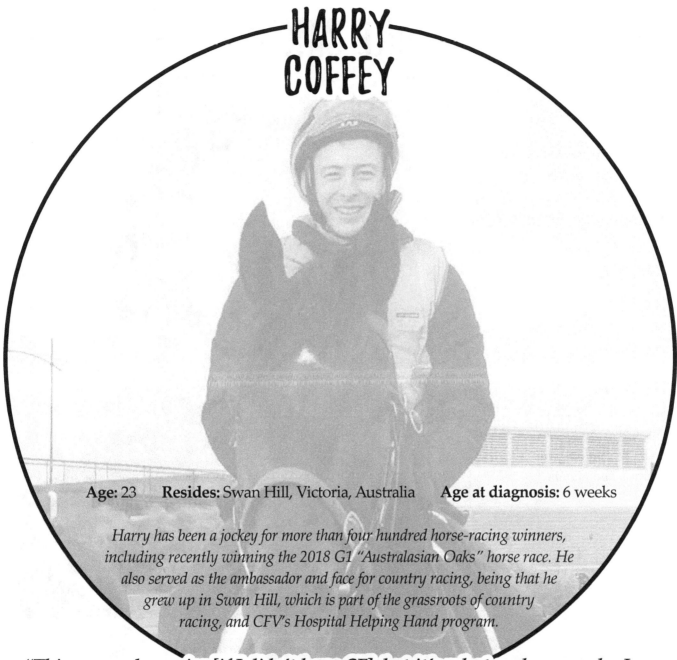

HARRY COFFEY

Age: 23   **Resides:** Swan Hill, Victoria, Australia   **Age at diagnosis:** 6 weeks

Harry has been a jockey for more than four hundred horse-racing winners, including recently winning the 2018 G1 "Australasian Oaks" horse race. He also served as the ambassador and face for country racing, being that he grew up in Swan Hill, which is part of the grassroots of country racing, and CFV's Hospital Helping Hand program.

"Things may be easier [if I didn't have CF], but it's what makes me who I am, and I am grateful for the person I am."

JAKE BAKER

Age: 17

Resides: Georgia, United States

Age at diagnosis: Before birth

First cadet with CF ever in the 111-year history of Riverside Military Academy; family has raised more than $6 million for the Cystic Fibrosis Foundation

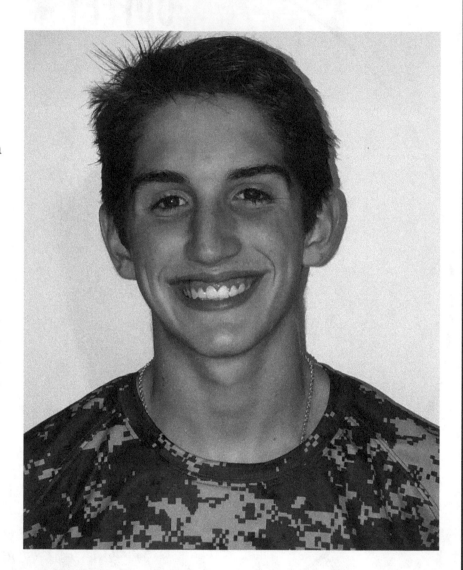

"But, I think the best thing that [CF] has done for me is it made me realize that I can endure hardships and overcome obstacles more than most people my age."

Jake Baker can literally say that people have been helping him in his fight against cystic fibrosis since before he was even born. While his mom, Pam, was pregnant with Jake, her son Gavin was diagnosed with CF at two years old. So, naturally, Jake was checked out and eventually diagnosed while Pam was six months pregnant with him. Neither of his two other siblings, Sabrina and Duncan, has cystic fibrosis.

"I wasn't very healthy for the first few years of my life," says Jake, who has spent a lot of time in the hospital. "My parents say that after a while, I was doing better, but I had a really hard time gaining weight."

As if the symptoms of the boys' disease weren't challenging enough, the financial cost of raising two boys requiring an extensive regimen of medications and therapies was prohibitive. Of course, Gavin and Jake's parents, Jon and Pam, weren't going down without a fight, so they rallied their family and friends to create their own army of soldiers that they named the Baker Boys' Battalion (BBB). "Although we had never raised a dime before," remembers Pam, "our army of soldiers raised over thirty thousand dollars that first year to become the number-one fundraising team in Georgia for the Great Strides Walk."

Now, almost seventeen years later, the BBB is still going strong, with teams all over the United States and Canada walking in Great Strides, hosting ShamRockin' For A Cure—their signature St. Patrick's Day parties in several states—biking Cycle for Life, driving Porches in their Smokies GT event, and playing in sporting events. Pam admits, "We have been so fortunate to have so many friends and even strangers who have now become such important members of our family. These warriors—our army of angels—have helped the BBB raise more than six million dollars for the Cystic Fibrosis Foundation so far!"

When Jake was ten, he got a feeding tube to help him gain some weight, primarily because his body mass index (BMI) was around 33 percent and he had not grown a centimeter in more than a year. Pam said she was very much in favor of it because, even though Jake was considered average weight (sixty-four pounds), she felt he was not growing at the rate that was expected based on the height potential of the family, and she was concerned he was not getting enough nutrition. Apparently, she was right. Jake gained about ten pounds a year for the three years he had the feeding tube.

Then, when Jake was in the sixth grade, he had his first official tune-up. "I was hospitalized for two weeks because my lung function kept going down," he says. "Being in the hospital wasn't so bad, though. My friends came to visit me, which was fun, and though it did get boring at times, I got to order room service whenever I wanted." While that might sound like the concerns of a typical kid, the truth was that Jake and Gavin badly needed treatments to improve their lung functions. The answer came in the form of a pill called Orkambi, which the FDA approved and gave "breakthrough therapy" status.

In August of 2015, Jake got his feeding tube removed about a week before he and his brother started their treatment of Orkambi. The Bakers had a huge party so that everyone who had helped them raise money over the years could watch Jake and Gavin take their very first dose. "It was so humbling that all of these people care about how long we live and how healthy we are!" says Jake. "We even played the *Rocky* theme song as we swallowed the pills. It was awesome!"

Jake knows that not everyone is blessed to have supportive parents like his. "I know that my parents will always fight for me and have my back, especially my mom. She's my champion, and her support for me is unending. I know that she and my dad will never stop trying to find a cure for everyone with cystic fibrosis."

And as far as Gavin goes, Jake says there are advantages and disadvantages to having a brother with CF. "We've heard of other people with CF who feel very lonely because they don't know anyone else with CF, but Gavin and I have always had each other. The hard part is we have to be really careful about not making each other sick. Our mom sharpies everything—our neb cups, our meds, our regular cups. We have to do our treatments in different rooms. So far, we haven't knowingly given anything to each other."

Maybe Jake's toughest hurdle has not been cystic fibrosis, but rather being able to reside at and attend a military school more than an hour northeast of the Bakers' suburban home. Jake has ADHD with a major emphasis on the impulsivity. Pam notes that Jake is extremely intelligent, but he was falling through the cracks in middle school and his grades were dropping considerably. Pam noticed that the "sparkle" had gone from his eyes.

Pam and Jon found Riverside Military Academy to be a much better fit for Jake, so they booked a tour. Jake loved it, and the school seemed to love him too . . . until they found out about his cystic fibrosis.

"I spoke with the infirmary and countered all of their objections," says Pam, who admits she was worried about sending her son away to school, but knew it was best for him. "I gathered information from the CF Foundation to build a case, and I got our admissions counselor on my side. So, he came up with a game plan to make it happen. Part of that game plan was to get the commandant on board with our plan, since he carried a lot of influence. So, operation 'win him over' was our next mission!"

Lieutenant Colonel (LTC) Spivey was the commandant of cadets, and had just joined the school a few months earlier after retiring from the army at the age of forty-four. He admits that he knew very little about CF, but he was very intrigued with Jake. "He reminded me of some of the recruits I had just seen when I left the army," he says. "The kid was a real go-getter and smart as a whip."

The school was still concerned about getting Jake in, but Pam believes that LTC Spivey was solely responsible for having them reconsider. "He agreed to take full responsibility of Jake's vest and breathing treatments, and keep all of it in his office and manage it himself! The infirmary agreed to handle all of his [pills], but none of the rest."

Thanks to LTC Spivey, Jake Baker became the first—and so far, the only—cadet with CF ever in the 111-year history of Riverside Military Academy.

LTC Spivey says, "Jake is essentially a normal kid, other than forty minutes in the morning and forty minutes in the evening when he comes in my office to do his treatments. He is not a threat to anyone here. He has single-handedly paved the way for the next kid with CF to get into Riverside Military Academy."

Jake is grateful for LTC Spivey's support. "He not only helped me get into Riverside, but he's helped me in so many ways that have nothing to do with CF. He is someone that I can go to with everyday troubles because I know that he'll listen and give me advice."

With Gavin departing last year for college, Jake is now a junior and an honor student at Riverside. He boasts a 4.17 GPA and has set a goal to get the highest grades in his class and someday attend MIT. He is also keeping up with all of his treatments and staying quite healthy. "Every day I have to do about three hours of physical exercise," he says. "Since I love tennis so much, I started a tennis club at school, so now I can spend those three hours playing tennis in the off-season. CF makes it very difficult at times to keep up with my teammates, but I keep doing it because I love it and it keeps me healthy. But, I think the best thing that [CF] has done for me is it made me realize that I can endure hardships and overcome obstacles more than most people my age."

LILY ROYER

Age: 19

Resides: Colorado, United States

Age at diagnosis: Just prior to her first birthday

Cofounder of Lilybart LLC; her story is featured in the February/ March 2019 issue of Mountain Parent *magazine, where Lilybart is the feature artist for all six covers of the magazine's 2019 editions; incoming freshman at University of Colorado Boulder in the fall of 2019*

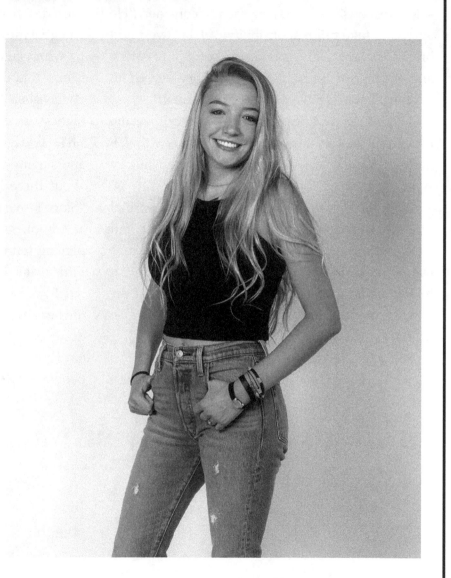

"I exercise at least three hours a day to stay ahead of the disease."

Most kids learn to take their first steps in the comfort of their own home. Lily Royer learned to walk pushing an IV pole down the halls of Columbia Hospital's pulmonary ward.

During her first year of life, a constant cough and poor digestion prevented Lily from gaining weight. After countless doctor visits with many different specialists, she was diagnosed with cystic fibrosis. Lily was admitted to Columbia University Medical Center in New York, where, over the course of two weeks, she underwent a battery of tests, surgeries, and treatments introducing her to a protocol of care for surviving CF.

Around the time Lily was in the third grade, her parents realized that she appeared most healthy and active every February when they visited the mountains of Colorado. So, they made the decision to relocate. "The decision was easy," says Lily's mom, Elana.

Lily's health definitely responded to the relocation. "We moved to the family ranch [in Aspen Valley]," Lily says. "I was hardly sick and began to catch up in height and weight."

Then, at fourteen years old, Lily was hospitalized with pneumonia. During this hospital stay, Lily's youngest brother, William, sent her a painting of a "really cool-looking heart." Everyone in the hospital who saw the painting said that it would make a great card. This diverted Lily's attention from the collapsed lung, as she and Elana printed the design on cardstock, distributed it to raise CF awareness, and then began to sketch out ideas for what would soon become Lilybart LLC, named after Lily's full name, Lillian Bartholomew Royer.

"Lilybart provides great opportunities for me to meet amazing and talented people who will always be in my life," says Lily, "and selling the cards allows me to tell my story and simultaneously raise awareness for cystic fibrosis." The money the company generates also helps Lily to augment the care that she receives at Children's Hospital Colorado to include acupuncture, massage, cupping, and chiropractic care.

Lily's uncanny organizational skills have allowed her to not just be the face of Lilybart, but to help run the business. "I have always been a very organized person," Lily says, "but I think having CF has made me that way. I have to keep track of my pills, my medicine, and make sure everything is always clean and sanitary."

Lily, who will be attending the University of Colorado Boulder in the fall of 2019, continues to make her card company and the foundation that goes along with it her biggest passions. Their purpose is to give other kids and young adults with CF a therapeutic outlet to exercise their creative passions, develop their skills through their collaborations with seasoned artists in both the Aspen Valley and Bucks County, Pennsylvania, regions, and raise money to help find a cure.

"I dream that a cure will be found soon," she says. "I want to have a family and travel the world."

BRYAN WARNECKE

Age: 20

Resides: Colorado, United States

Age at diagnosis: 3 weeks

Biked 1,065 miles over forty-three days to help raise $300,000 for the Cystic Fibrosis Center at Children's Colorado; star of the OneRepublic music video "I Lived," which has been seen by nearly forty million people

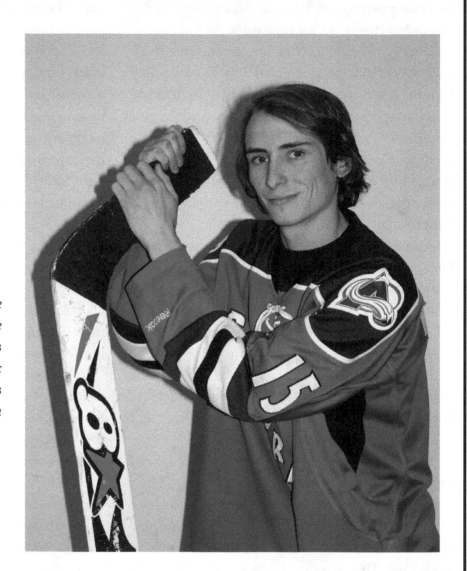

"I am living my dreams, owning every second this world could give, and I know that when my moment comes, I will be able to say, 'I did it all!'"

"I did it all" are the poignant lyrics of OneRepublic's song "I Lived." Who would think that someone born with cystic fibrosis could one day be the centerpiece for those words? Meet Bryan Warnecke.

Bryan was born to teenagers not yet ready to raise a family. This opened the door to parenthood for two loving adoptive parents who so badly wanted to expand their family, despite health issues that precluded mom, Wendy, from having another child herself.

The family was so incredibly happy when they received the call that one of the adoption agency's birth mothers had chosen their family for her soon-to-be-born son. However, during the first three weeks of Bryan's life, food would pass quickly through him. He failed to gain weight, and Steve and Wendy were up with him nearly every hour feeding him and changing his diapers. At three weeks, they took him back to Children's Hospital Colorado for more tests to find out what was wrong, and were told that he had cystic fibrosis.

Bryan made nineteen trips to and spent thirty nights in the hospital his first six months. Wendy remembers those first months as the most difficult of her life. "I was there in the hospital with Bryan, sleeping in the recliner next to his bed so that I was never more than a few steps away," she says.

Bryan seemed to get healthier after that and settled into twice-daily treatments and multiple medications, including enzymes with all food. Not only did he thrive, Wendy and Steve say he learned to run before he could walk.

At two years old, after watching the neighborhood boys playing street hockey, Bryan strapped on his brother's skates. When his mother reminded him that he did not know how to skate, he replied, "You just stand up and go!" The neighborhood boys strapped goalie gear onto Bryan and were thrilled to have someone in front of the net. Little did they know what they had started; Bryan's hockey career was born.

At six years old, Bryan began playing organized rec inline hockey. He was so good that when his older brother's team needed a goalie because theirs was going to be out of town, Bryan stepped in and played against kids four years older than him.

At eight, Bryan stepped onto the ice for the first time wearing pink goalie pads—a fact that led his goalie coach to give him the name "Pink Lightning," which has stuck to this day. Bryan's teammates loved it. Opposing players made fun until the game started and Bryan shut them up with his play. He was the only goalie for the team that year, and led them to the championship and several tournament wins around the state of Colorado. He would occasionally do a respiratory treatment at the rink, and the other kids would ask him about it, but none of them treated Bryan any differently. All they knew was that despite the issues that compelled these treatments, he "did it all."

Then, at age fifteen, in the weeks leading up to

the state championship tournament, Bryan became increasingly sick. Though he missed a lot of school, he never missed a practice or game. Bryan was able to play in the state tournament and share time with another goalie. Partway into the second period of the championship game, the team was down three to two. Bryan came in, stopped seventeen shots over the course of the rest of the game, and his team won the championship 5–4.

Bryan was the hero of his high school team, but no one knew how much he went through to get there. That night, with the season over, his body collapsed. He had a fever from a respiratory infection, and spent the next two days in bed before his parents checked him into Children's Hospital Colorado for a week. This was the first time that Bryan had been hospitalized since he was a baby, and it was a reality check for the family that CF was real and ever-progressing.

While lying in the hospital bed with his dad at his side, Bryan felt run down, out of energy, and his lung function declined. Anybody would understand if he needed a break from thinking about CF, but that was not Bryan. The two dreamed up a bike tour throughout Colorado called the Pink Lightning Tour to raise money and awareness for the Cystic Fibrosis Center at Children's Hospital Colorado.

They trained for a few months and planned the route. They also developed a website to help them raise funds for the cause. Their journey began in June of 2014 in a very visible SUV wrapped in pink lightning bolts. The route started at Children's Hospital in Denver and finished at the Courage Classic in Copper Mountain. In total, they rode their bikes 1,065 miles over forty-three days that summer through forty-six Colorado towns and over eight mountain passes.

The ride began with thirty riders, with participants changing as the locales did, but Bryan and Steve were the only two to ride the entire way. They raised $300,000 for the Cystic Fibrosis Center at Children's Colorado, and the media picked up the story everywhere that they went. They managed to do the Cystic Cycle for Life in the years following in other cities around the US to benefit the Cystic Fibrosis Foundation. Steve estimates they raised a grand total of $700,000 for cystic fibrosis research.

While all of this was going on, OneRepublic band leader Ryan Tedder mentioned to his friend Colorado Governor John Hickenlooper that the band was looking for the right story to tell in the video for their single "I Lived." Governor Hickenlooper referred Tedder to the CEO of Children's Hospital, Jim Shmerling, who was very familiar with Bryan and his story.

"Let me tell you about Bryan Warnecke," said CEO Shmerling, who proceeded to tell Tedder Bryan's story. Tedder loved the idea because Bryan exemplified the message of the song, which is living life to its fullest despite the obstacles.

"The song is Bryan," says Steve.

Bryan can be seen in the video "living his life"

with cystic fibrosis. Nearly forty million people have now seen it, and thousands of messages have come from around the world thanking Bryan for reminding people of how life should be lived.

Bryan's career as a public face of CF took off from the video. After the bike tour and music video, the Colorado Avalanche, Denver's NHL franchise, invited Bryan to skate the pregame skate before their NHL game. He also spoke to the audience of nearly twenty thousand people after showing the "I Lived" video.

Then, at seventeen years old, Bryan's life turned. "I began smoking marijuana. Even worse, I stopped doing the CF treatments, was only partially compliant with my meds, and was vaping. I had lived with CF, the meds, the treatments, and all that goes along with it for seventeen years, and I just wanted to be a normal teenager doing normal teenage things. Unfortunately, this was a very unhealthy combination for someone with a lung disease, and while in the hospital, my doctor told me, 'If you keep treating your body like this, you will be dead within a year.'"

Bryan, whom his family knew would have a better chance to thrive in a physical-rehabilitation facility in the wilderness, landed at Open Sky Wilderness in the mountains of southwestern Colorado and the Canyonlands of Utah. Open Sky embraced the complexities of CF that Bryan presented, and made many accommodations to facilitate his participation. Bryan had only a sleeping bag, tarp, and backpack, no access to running water or electricity, and lived in the wilderness with his support group.

Seventy-one days after entering Open Sky and right before his eighteenth birthday, Bryan graduated from the program and returned to the "real" world. He is committed to his new healthy lifestyle and remains clean and sober to this day, returning to regular CF treatments and meds. "I knew I had to pull myself out of my downward spiral very quickly and turn my life around," says Bryan. "I am healthy and happy again."

Says Steve, "Bryan is still a young man with all that goes with that, including some things that aren't perfect for his health. He is not perfectly compliant with CF treatments, but is making the effort and is better at it. His lungs show some damage from the last few years, but he hasn't had a recent hospitalization."

In May 2018, Brian graduated from high school. Today, he is helping other kids deal with their addictions and is looking forward to resuming speaking, telling his story, and motivating others to live life to its fullest. "I am living my dreams," he says, "owning every second this world could give, and I know that when my moment comes, I will be able to say, 'I did it all!'"

MATT MITCHELL

Age: 21

Resides: Arizona, United States

Age at diagnosis: 3 days

Recipient of the National Football Foundation (NFF) National Scholar Athlete award; recipient of the Bear award at Phoenix College, awarded to the best student athlete of the year for all sports at the school; co-offensive most-valuable player (MVP) at Phoenix College, and Arizona Junior College Scholar Athlete of the Year; currently serving on the CF Family Advisory Council at Phoenix Children's Hospital

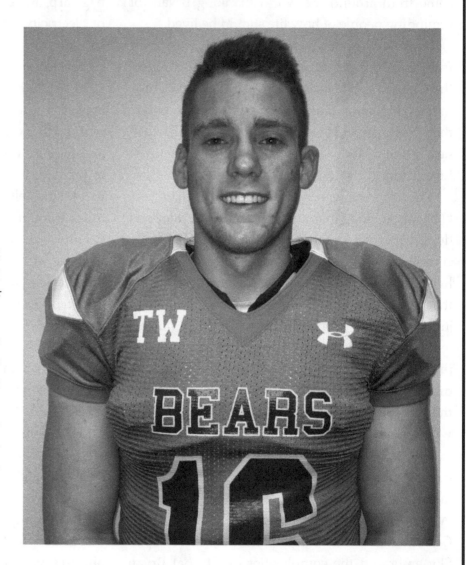

"[Playing Division I football] would then give me a platform where I can help others with CF and inspire them to pursue their dreams while raising awareness."

Matt Mitchell has been scoring touchdowns for years, but it's his off-field story that has people talking.

When Matt was born, he looked like a happy and healthy baby, according to his father, Tom. "He was pink, alert, and energetic with no difficulties. He was twenty-one inches tall and weighed eight pounds and six ounces." Yet, when it came time to feed Matt, his parents saw that he couldn't hold down any food. He was moved to the nursery around ten hours after birth, and then to the pediatric ICU four hours later for closer observation. After a couple of x-rays and an examination, they decided to do an exploratory abdominal surgery to figure out what was wrong. The doctor came out from the procedure and told his parents that Matt had meconium ileus that was 95 percent indicative of cystic fibrosis.

At three days old, Matt started his CF treatment routine of taking sprinkled enzymes with applesauce and percussion by hand a couple of times daily. A month later, the DNA test confirmed the diagnosis.

He started on the vest at age three. "My parents set it up on a chair in their room and hooked my first video game up to their TV," says Matt. "The best thing my parents did for me was making treatment something I wanted to do. The only time I could play video games was during treatment, and that always made it exciting for me."

But Matt's parents also made sure he was very active at a young age, playing all kinds of sports. As he got older and more disciplined with his conditioning, nutrition, and weight gain, Matt's focus on sports switched to only football. "I trained day in and day out, and stayed on top of my meals so I could keep my weight up with everybody else. In eighth grade, I started lifting seriously and saw leaps in strength and size like none of my peers, because CF had made me disciplined, and that carried over to how I ate and trained."

Matt worked extremely hard and started his sophomore year on varsity as receiver and backed up their senior quarterback. His junior season, he earned the starting quarterback spot—all while his coaches knew nothing of his CF. "I had a great season and felt I had proved I could really play at the top," says Matt. "That is when I agreed to come out with my story about playing with cystic fibrosis."

When it came out, Matt didn't expect all the appreciation he received. Coaches and peers respected him for all that he'd accomplished despite the battle. Matt reassured those that were worried that he was okay, and explained a little bit more about the disease. "It was hard initially to come out of my shell about [CF] because I tended to keep that part of my life private, and we didn't want coaches to fear it and restrict me, rather than push me to be my best. Previously, anytime I took enzymes at school, I just said they were pills I had to take to help my digestion and left it at that. After the story came out, I quickly came to realize I had an opportunity to not only inspire, but to inform people on what the disease is and what CF patients deal with daily."

Going into his training for his senior year, Matt was more motivated than ever. He had done track in the spring semester of his junior year, and won state in the 4x100 meter relay. He eventually maxed out at a 325-pound bench, a 455-pound squat, and a 265-pound power clean at the end of his junior year. He trained day in and day out all summer heading into his senior year. He was waking up at 4:45 a.m. for 5:30 a.m. workouts with a flexibility-and-speed coach, lifting later in the day with his team, and then throwing with his quarterback coach to touch up on his form and accuracy. He'd try to be in bed early to enhance his recovery. "As long as I had proper rest, I felt great throughout my workouts. I'd have a bit of a cough after running a lot, but it only helped me clear my lungs and be ready for the next workout."

That fall, Matt led his team to a 13–0 state championship season with three thousand passing yards, nine hundred rushing yards, forty-five passing touchdowns, twelve rushing touchdowns, and only two interceptions. He finished remarkably with the fourth-best quarterback rating in the nation.

Matt questioned whether Division I schools were more hesitant to recruit him because he was only 5'8", which was far from ideal for a college quarterback, or because of his cystic fibrosis. He eventually found the right fit and was given an opportunity to showcase his football skills as a wide receiver at Phoenix College, a junior college in Arizona. Upon returning to the field his freshman year, Matt had a touchdown reception and threw a touchdown pass. Going into his sophomore season, he was voted team captain by his teammates.

Matt has since sprouted a few more inches to 5'10.5". After finishing his sophomore season at Phoenix College, where he was the co-offensive MVP, Matt was recruited as a walk-on receiver for the University of Arizona after a camp performance in late June 2018. Matt is a pre-med student and will be part of the team roster when practice starts in the spring of 2019. Matt knows that playing at the next level will do more than just improve the competition he faces. "It would then give me a platform where I can help others with CF," he says, "and inspire them to pursue their dreams while raising awareness."

That will be Matt's greatest score.

MURIELLE TIERNAN

Age: 24   **Resides:** Virginia, United States   **Age at diagnosis:** 6 months

Murielle is the career record holder for most goals, multigoal games, game winners, and points in Virginia Tech Hokie soccer history, a three-year first-team All-Atlantic Coast Conference (ACC) selection, and a member of the 2013 Hokie team that competed in the College Cup (the final four of Women's NCAA Division I soccer). After graduating from Virginia Tech in 2017, Murielle is now playing soccer overseas in Stockholm, Sweden, for Hammarby IF of the Damallsvenskan league, the top professional league in Sweden.

"My attitude in dealing with treatments influenced my attitude on the field."

OWEN WRIGHT

Age: 22

Resides: Massachusetts, United States

Age at diagnosis: 2 months

Atlantic 10 All-Conference in the 800 Free Relay and owner of the school record in the 200 IM his freshman year at UMass; Atlantic 10 First Team All-Conference honors in the 200 free relay and 800 free relay; Atlantic 10 Second Team All-Conference honors in the 400 free relay his sophomore year at UMass; undefeated in the 50 freestyle in the Atlantic 10 regular season his senior year at UMass; UMass school record holder in the 50 free and the 200, 400, and 800 free relays and 400 medley relay

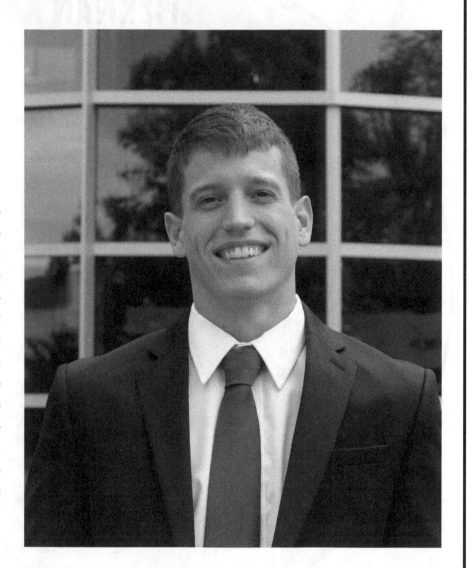

"I'm a very competitive person by nature. With or without CF, I'd still be the athlete I am today."

Thirteen-time Atlantic 10 Conference (A-10) Coach of the Year Russ Yarworth, head coach at the University of Massachusetts Amherst (UMass) for nearly four decades, kept hearing about a record-breaking swimmer named Owen Wright from his hometown of Attleboro, Massachusetts. Owen was a three-year letter winner at Attleboro High School. He was the 2013 Massachusetts State Champion in the 50 and 200 freestyle events, and was named the 2012–2013 All-Scholastic Swimmer of the Year by the *Boston Globe* and *Boston Herald*.

Yarworth finally had the opportunity to return to his hometown to meet Owen and his parents during Owen's senior year. That's when Coach Yarworth got the full story. Owen's father, Vern, asked his son to reveal his health situation. Russ said he did a double take when he found out that Owen had CF, but that didn't stop him from pursuing the young man to swim at UMass.

"I didn't look at it as a negative," says Yarworth. "This kid's gonna be tough. He's gonna be able to swim. He's gonna be able to give it."

Owen didn't want to let his coach down. "I was worried that Russ thought I would get sick, which could happen, but staying on top of everything has taught me a lot."

Growing up, Owen's parents, Kat and Vern, were very adamant that Owen live outside the dreaded "CF bubble." Owen says the best thing his parents did was not make a big deal about the disease and treating him like his other record-breaking swimming siblings, seventeen-year-old brother River and fourteen-year-old sister Brynn. Neither of his siblings has CF.

"'You're a great athlete, Owen,' they would say to me. 'Go out and get it.'"

Owen began realizing the severity of CF early on in high school when he cultured pseudomonas and later, in his college career, when he required an extended hospital stay with other critically ill people. "This was not a joke." He soon found an elixir for the concerns of CF. "I escaped my fear through exercise. I am always outrunning something."

Owen started swimming in eighth grade more for fun than anything else. In ninth grade he started getting competitive as a member of the Attleboro Bluefish Swim Club (ABS), an elite swim club in New England. It requires roughly three to four hours a day between morning and afternoon practices, seven days a week, while most clubs require five to six days a week with fewer committed hours. Owen says that his experience at Bluefish helped his confidence. "I knew I could handle D1 athletics and knew I could back up my narrative as a solid athlete who hasn't let the disease throw him off."

Swimming has been Owen's main form of airway clearance for years. He only does vest treatments when he is sick, along with antibiotics. He says that oral antibiotics have been very beneficial for him, and only twice has he had to use IV antibiotics. He also regularly takes enzymes with meals to help with digestion.

Coach Yarworth says, "Owen has 'go juice.' He loves to race. He has a tremendous motor. He's motivated."

Owen adds, "I'm a very competitive person by nature. With or without CF, I'd still be the athlete I am today."

Owen had a great four-year career at UMass, but it was in his senior year in 2017–2018 that he defied logic and denied CF with his performances. He had the best competition season of his life. He says he committed himself to eating better and staying as healthy as possible, and it paid off. He won almost every race. He was even sick at some of the meets, including the last dual meet held at his home pool, the final meet that his family was able to attend. Owen took advantage. He set two pool records at the 50 free and 100 free at that meet while dealing with a staph infection in his lungs requiring oral antibiotics.

Coach Yarworth reflects on Owen's amazing career. "My own opinion is that the competitiveness in which he fights the disease certainly manifests itself in the competitiveness in which he approached competition."

Owen, whose motto is "Live in the present with enthusiasm for success," explains that he has to put in more effort than others who may not have the disease who are competing against him.

Owen graduated in the fall of 2018 with a degree in economics. While this D1 athlete no longer swims for UMass, the Massachusetts native can still boast of an FEV1 of 101 percent while "swimming laps" around the disease that has been challenging his lungs since the day he was born.

BOBBY FOSTER

Age: 25 **Resides:** Florida, United States **Age at diagnosis:** Birth

Bobby is a spoken-word poet, storyteller, and life coach. A graduate of the University of Central Florida, Bobby was on the school's Poetry Slam Team, which placed in one of the top positions at the College Unions Poetry Slam Invitational (CUPSI), one of the most prestigious collegiate spoken-word contests in the world. His Facebook spoken-word videos have reached over a million views around the world. Bobby's book Catch Your Breath *shows readers that they have "the power to create the lives they want to live." The young Floridian recently received a CF Impact Grant from the Cystic Fibrosis Foundation so that he, as a life coach, can take on clients with CF for free for a three-month period.*

"I'm working on being able to be productive and efficient even while I feel sick, and cherishing the moments when I don't."

TEENA MOBLEY

Age: 23

Resides: New York, United States

Age at diagnosis: 9

Ranked third in the national rankings of the National Junior College Athletic Association (NJCAA), with her best jump being measured at 19'6" in the long jump while at Monroe College

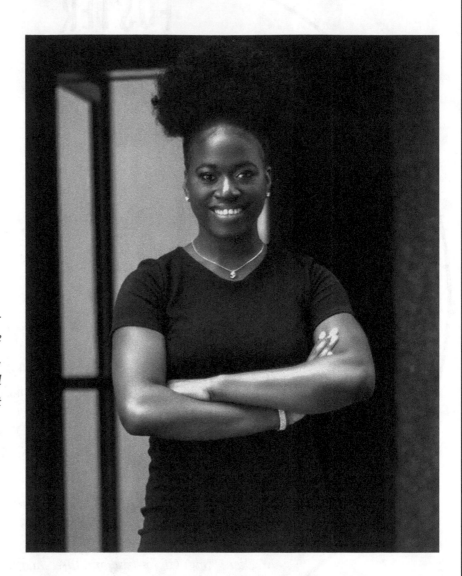

"I plan to overcome my obstacles by keeping a positive mindset, being a hard worker, being a role model for others as well as helping them, and to just be great."

Born from a drug-addicted and alcoholic mother, Teena was adopted and brought into the Mobley family through foster care when she was twenty-one months old, along with her two little brothers. She grew up in Long Island, New York, and always had a passion for sports. "Especially basketball and track," she says.

Despite being athletic, Teena had issues that no one seemed to have answers for. She would sweat a lot, and the sweat was very salty. She also tired often, even from just walking a set of stairs. She had difficulty gaining weight, and was in and out of the hospital regularly because she was often sick. Her doctors blamed it on asthma—until the moment when everything changed.

"One day after playing basketball with my neighbors, I started to feel really weird and sick. It was very hard for me to breathe. I kept coughing." After this latest attack, Teena's parents no longer accepted the asthma diagnosis. She was once again hospitalized, and her symptoms became worse. "My chest was tight. I didn't have a lot of fat on my body to fight off the sickness. I was just lying there with my eyes closed."

Soon, the answer was revealed. At the age of nine, she was diagnosed with cystic fibrosis. "This experience made a drastic change in my life," she says. "I was hospitalized to the point that the hospital felt like home. The doctors told my parents that I may not make it, and for some reason, I didn't really know what that meant. Or maybe I did know, but was in denial about lying on my deathbed. My parents were so heartbroken that I was misdiagnosed with asthma and that I had almost passed away that night in the hospital."

She remembers her mom screaming, "We could have lost her! We could have lost her!" upon finding out that Teena had CF.

Life-saving measures allowed her to walk out of the hospital on this occasion, but soon after, the significance of the diagnosis started to set in. "When I slowly started to recover," says Teena, "I was taking a bunch of medications, went through many tests, and was given treatments. Due to the CF diagnosis, I was told that my capabilities would be fairly limited." Then, it hit her. "I thought my dream of being a competitive athlete was over."

She was not going down without a fight.

Coming out of high school, Teena was awarded All Long Island as New York State's top long jumper in track and field, her maximum jump being an astounding 18'9". She graduated with other athletic honors, including All County for Suffolk County and MVP of her high school team, which was voted on by her teammates.

Teena received a track scholarship from Monroe College in New Rochelle, New York, where she attended for two years, balancing her studies and CF treatments while also being one of the top long jumpers in the nation and an All-American 4x4 meter relay competitor. Still, it was not easy for Teena. She had to be sure to eat the right foods and keep up with her treatment regimen, which began every morning at 4:30 a.m. "I had to work way harder than others, but I managed to finish my workouts and keep a strong mentality. When I would train, I wouldn't have it in my mind that I have a breathing illness. CF would not be a reason that I couldn't compete or train."

After obtaining her associate's degree in business administration from Monroe, she received a track-and-field scholarship to Long Island University Brooklyn, an NCAA Division I school.

"Being a track athlete and competing at a D1 level is beneficial to me because I am getting the right amount of exercise my body needs to help manage my cystic fibrosis," says Teena. "The training also helps improve my breathing and makes my heart stronger. Training and competing has helped me see my overall potential. I may have to work a little harder than everyone, but that does not mean that I cannot do what others can do. I do not let my illness control me or get to me mentally."

Teena wants others to know that they are more than capable of repeating her accomplishments.

"One of my main goals was to inspire others, and by me competing at a D1 level, that shows people that anything is possible if you put your mind to it. If you have a dream, then go for it.

"There are times when I am in pain and there are days that my breathing is better than another day," she continues, "but I always remained aware that although I have this illness, I am as physically fit and mentally strong-minded as I think someone can be considering my circumstances."

Teena balanced six classes and two internships while trying to manage being an athlete. Her greatest accomplishment, she says, was managing a 3.5 GPA throughout college while training for and competing annually in the Penn Relays, the US's oldest and largest track-and-field event.

"Could you imagine how exhausted I am most of the time?" she says in mock exasperation. "At the end of the day, though, I know my limits, and I feel like it will all pay off in the end. I plan to overcome my obstacles by keeping a positive mindset, being a hard worker, being a role model for others as well as helping them, and to just be great."

SOPHIE GRACE HOLMES

Age: 27   **Resides:** London, England, United Kingdom   **Age at diagnosis:** 4 months

Sophie, a fitness model, personal trainer, and avid exercise enthusiast, has accomplished several incredible athletic feats to raise funds for the CF Trust. Most notably, she climbed 19,341 feet to the top of Mount Kilimanjaro in October 2015, 15,777 feet to the top of Mont Blanc in July 2018, and trekked 14,763 feet of the Himalayas in October 2018.

"I feel my CF has made me the person I am. I am lucky to have the life I have, and I am determined to keep fighting and to enjoy every minute."

33

JASON VAN'T SLOT

Age: 24

Resides: Cape Town, Western Cape, South Africa

Age at diagnosis: 8 months

Competitive mountain-bike racer and road cyclist; world's first person with CF to complete the Cape Epic (2015); world's first person with CF to ride a sub three-hour Cape Town Cycle Tour (2018)

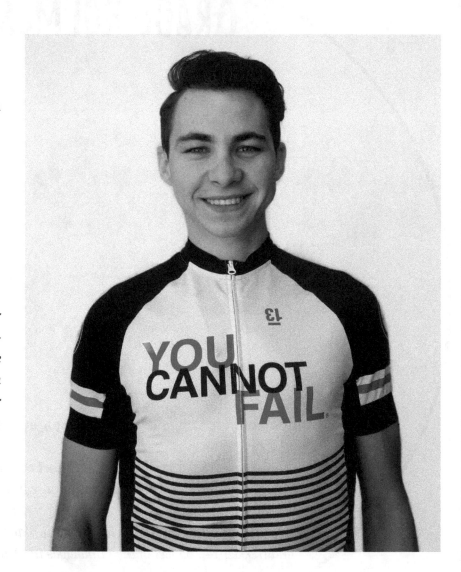

"My father told me that I was never allowed to use cystic fibrosis as an excuse."

vid mountain biker Jason van't Slot and his twin sister, Carla, were born on February 10, 1995, in South Africa. As a baby, Jason wasn't putting on any weight despite drinking liters of milk. He was taken to three different pediatricians, but none could figure out what was wrong. When Jason was eight months old, after various lung infections, often being constipated, and still failing to thrive, Jason's family wanted answers. A family friend, Dr. Clive Tucker, who was also a general practitioner, saw he was blue in the face and insisted Jason be sent to the hospital to undergo a sweat test. Dr. Tucker suspected that CF may be the culprit, because being blue in the face meant a lack of oxygen. He sent Jason and his family to Life Vincent Pallotti Hospital in Cape Town and wrote a note to the doctor there outlining what Jason had previously experienced and why he suggested a sweat test. That day, Jason was diagnosed with cystic fibrosis, and his family was told that living beyond the age of ten was virtually impossible.

When Jason was three years old, his father punished him because "I said I couldn't do something because I was sick. My father told me that I was never allowed to use cystic fibrosis as an excuse." That punishment may have been an extremely hard thing for his father to give, but Jason is now thankful, as the message was the building block to how he has lived his life.

As a young child, Jason was taught that everyone has something to deal with; it is just a matter of accepting it and getting on with life in the best way possible. "It is easy for a young child to say, 'Why me?' But, I never asked that question, as I felt that it had no real meaning. We have a family motto that says, 'Don't give it power,' implying that something can't control you if you don't give it the power to do so." As a means to diminish its power and control, Jason only refers to cystic fibrosis by the abbreviation "CF" whenever possible.

As a teen, Jason never had the urge to research online what CF actually was. "I knew the basics," he says, "and that I had it, but I was completely oblivious to the implications or the fact that CF is life-threatening. I never felt the need to know more. It was just something that I have, but it wasn't who I was. I think by not exposing myself to the stories of others on the internet. It has helped me to not put a targeted life expectancy like most people with CF."

In 2010, when Jason was around the age of fifteen, he and his father rode the 109 kilometers (60 miles) of the Cape Town Cycle Tour as a bucket-list activity that all Cape Townians must do. "I thought it would be my last and only Cape Town Cycle Tour. My dad explained the finer points of cycling and strategies throughout the tour. After being injured with a torn ligament in my ankle from playing soccer a year earlier, he suggested I join him for one of his Sunday rides, as it was less taxing on my ankle. In true van't Slot fashion of go big or go home, he took me on a sixty-kilometer

(37.2 miles) trek, which left me completely broken and crying five kilometers from home."

Instead of wanting to quit, Jason's passion for the sport emerged. He was out the next weekend doing the same route and feeling much stronger. Soon, he was joining his dad and his friends every weekend.

"He set up a training program for me at the 2012 Cape Town Cycle Tour, where I cut two hours and forty minutes off our time from 2010. I was so disappointed with myself for not breaking the four-hour mark by five minutes. The next year I cut a further fifty minutes off my time." Still, Jason wanted to eventually cut that time even more. The day before completing his first tour in 2010, Jason promised his father that he would someday be one of the small percentage of amateur riders who could do a "sub 3." That means doing the race in under three hours.

Jason's ultimate goal was to ride the Cape Epic, a Western Cape–based competitive mountain-biking stage race where the actual route of the race is not released until the night before the event. The Cape Epic is widely renowned as the toughest mountain-bike race in the world; Jason calls it the mountain-biking version of the Tour de France. It is the equivalent of almost riding the height of Mount Everest twice in eight hundred kilometers. Any rider who completes the Cape Epic is considered to have achieved a huge accomplishment in the cycling community, as it is raced by elite athletes from all over the world who see this race as the ultimate challenge. The big-picture obstacle, of course, was staying healthy enough to be in the position to simply consider such an extreme event. Jason's goal was to ride it in 2015.

The reality of managing the training demands and competitive schedule for a race such as the Cape Epic didn't disappoint. Generally, he had to watch his health very closely so as not to get sick in the five months leading up to the event. In terms of his day-to-day, he had to monitor his heart rate every morning and evening to determine if he needed that extra day of recovery typical for a cyclist, and relieve hemoptysis episodes while out training by taking short breaks whenever they occurred. Fortunately, when he has had hemoptysis episodes during races, they were small enough for him not to have to stop, they clotted pretty quickly, and after spitting blood out once or twice, he was good to go. Jason said he had some nastier episodes during his training, but knew to either tone it down or head home in order to prevent it from becoming worse.

His can-do attitude translates to how he sees himself in the CF community. "As cliché as it all sounds," he says, "I always knew that I would one day inspire or teach others that it is not the circumstances that you are born in, it is what you do with those circumstances that defines who you are. I felt that I could show the parents of young children with this disease that CF doesn't have to be a death sentence. Their child can still participate in competitive sports like I have. It is a mindset, and therefore they must not convince their child that they can't accomplish their goals."

In 2015, a year after he competed in the Cape Country MTB Tour, Jason entered the Cape Epic with his teammate and close friend Philipp Sassie. "Our goal was to ride the Cape Epic for charity and raise awareness and funds for the Cape Cystic Fibrosis Association, which supports the Red Cross Children's Hospital. It would be a thank-you for all of their support throughout my life."

In order to compete in the Cape Epic, a participant has to be at least nineteen and must have a full medical checkup before taking part. Amongst the 1,300 riders are amateurs like Jason, Olympians, and even world champions.

"In an attempt to portray CF more positively, we named our team Cystic Fibrosis Cycling RSA with the motto 'Breathing in life' rather than the destructive motto of CF South Africa's 'We fight to breathe.' We were not trying to portray that I was a CF cyclist, but rather a cyclist who happened to have CF."

On March 22, 2015, at the age of twenty, Jason, along with Philipp, became the first team to complete the Cape Epic with a rider with CF.

Jason got a lot of media coverage for his work at the Cape Epic. He was featured in online articles and print magazines, did some radio interviews, and was even asked to be a keynote speaker at several events.

In 2018, at the age of twenty-three, Jason burst into tears as he kept his long-awaited promise to his father and finally accomplished his "sub 3." He became the first person with CF to complete the Cape Town Cycle Tour in under three hours after eight years of pursuing this unique achievement.

Having a chronic disease may kill the average person's spirit, but it has done the opposite for Jason van't Slot. "It has allowed me to believe in the impossible."

ANGELA DESTASIO

Age: 25

Resides: New Jersey, United States

Age at diagnosis: 8 months

Graduated from the prestigious dance program at Marymount Manhattan College; performed in Train, a production by famed choreographer Robert Battle, at the Theresa Long Theatre in New York City in January 2016; dance instructor; 2017–2019 NBA dancer for the Philadelphia 76ers; 2018–2019 dance team cocaptain for the Philadelphia 76ers

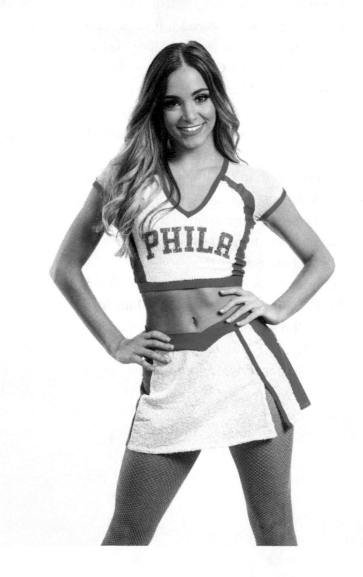

"I started to realize I aspired to dance for my whole life. It isn't a concrete future, but nobody with CF knows what a concrete future is."

Angela DeStasio grew up with the scary CF prognosis, but her mindset has always been strong. "You have to put yourself first, mentally and physically. You can attain any goal you want. Take care of your mind just as much as your lungs."

Angela was hospitalized more than a dozen times during her childhood, starting in second grade from a lung exacerbation. She calls her tune-up in seventh grade, during which she was stuck in the hospital with pneumonia and told, along with her parents, that she may not make it out, her worst CF memory. At seventeen, she had her first experience with hemoptysis. "I was lying on my bed watching TV. I felt a kind of bubbling in my chest that felt foreign. I sat up and coughed into my hand and noticed blood splattered onto my palm. I ran to the bathroom sink and it started coming up. My mom heard me and ran to my side through it all. It was scary."

Angela survived the frightening CF experiences throughout her youth and found inspiration in two forms: modern dance, and her best friend and big sister, Melissa—currently thirty-four, a devoted wife, mom of two, former pediatric nurse . . . and a CF patient.

Despite her challenges with CF—she tells friends in her improvisation class to breathe out of a straw while holding their noses and dancing at the same time in order to "get a feel" for how she feels while she is dancing—and once-a-year tune-ups, she was accepted to the prestigious dance program at Marymount Manhattan College. She graduated with not just a major in dance, but a minor in psychology that Angela used to better understand children in her quest to become a dance teacher.

Angela now teaches and uses that platform to raise awareness. "I absolutely love being a dance teacher. While my initial dream was to be a professional dancer, I started to realize I aspired to something even bigger—to dance for my whole life. It isn't a concrete future, but nobody with CF knows what a concrete future is." Nevertheless, her career grew dance legs, and in January of 2016 Angela performed in *Train* at the Theresa Lang Theatre in New York City.

In 2017, Angela's busy life became busier and more exciting when she was selected to become a member of the official dance team of the NBA's Philadelphia 76ers that performs at all forty-one home games. "It is the greatest job. Getting to do community work as a team and perform almost every day for crowds of twenty thousand people is indescribable." Angela increased her role the following season, as she was named cocaptain.

As for how CF fits into Angela's life, she makes sure fighting CF is her number-one priority. "Exercise is part of my profession, so that keeps my lungs in great shape, and I do my treatments in the morning and at night, so my job doesn't get in the way of my health."

REID D'AMICO

Age: 26

Resides: Maryland, United States

Age at diagnosis: 10

Biomedical engineer at US Food and Drug Administration (FDA); director of the US Adult Cystic Fibrosis Association; National Science Foundation Graduate Research fellow; recipient of the Cystic Fibrosis Scholarship Foundation and Boomer Esiason Foundation scholarships; science-and-research columnist with BioNews Services; *columnist with* CF News; *earned his PhD in the summer of 2018*

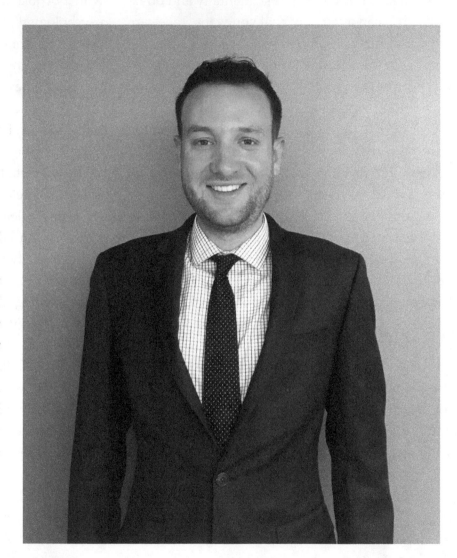

"I am always excited to work with companies and foundations in the CF community because this is the best way to make sure that the voices of those with CF are heard."

Some people do not want to be defined by CF, but Dr. Reid D'Amico has found his life's calling in it. "By being an engineer in a medical field," he says, "I'm able to apply various engineering techniques to better understand, model, treat, and diagnose disease."

Reid was born outside of Washington, DC, but spent the majority of his childhood in Hilton Head Island, South Carolina. It took the doctors ten long years before they could finally diagnose Reid with CF after discovering nasal polyps during one of his colds. "I was young," he says, recalling the diagnosis, "but I remember the doctor bluntly telling my parents while I was in the room how many of life's milestones (graduations, marriage, etc.) would never happen for me."

Reid says that his CF diagnosis forced him to rethink his priorities as a teenager. "Instead of dirty locker rooms, I put more time into academics. I have been fascinated with medical research, and specifically rare lung diseases."

Reid attended Duke University in Durham, North Carolina, and majored in biomedical engineering, focusing the majority of his undergraduate research on stem cells, tissue engineering, and regenerative medicine. He graduated from Duke in May of 2015, and immediately started his PhD in biomedical engineering at Vanderbilt University in Nashville, Tennessee.

Reid's ultimate goal is to create a career researching and advocating for cystic fibrosis. "I am always excited to work with companies and foundations in the CF community because this is the best way to make sure that the voices of those with CF are heard. I am grateful of all of these opportunities, and am looking forward to influencing the CF community by increasing my contribution to those with the disease." Reid also wants to be able to help CF patients by helping them afford medication.

Reid has found that volunteering and getting involved with people with all kinds of diseases helped him find a purpose. His advice? Use your story to make a difference for others. "Having CF gives you a powerful story," he says. "Make sure you share it. Finding time to help others gives you a sense of purpose, and ultimately leads to greater motivation in life."

MICHAEL ROWE

Age: 27

Resides: Colorado, United States

Age at diagnosis: 23

The only CF patient known to climb all fifty-eight of Colorado's 14ers; climbed to the top of the Andes' Aconcagua in the Mendoza Province, Argentina, and Mount Kilimanjaro in Tanzania, Africa; climbed a total of one hundred different 13er summits in Colorado and a grand total (including repeat trips) of close to two hundred summits of over 13,000 feet within the state

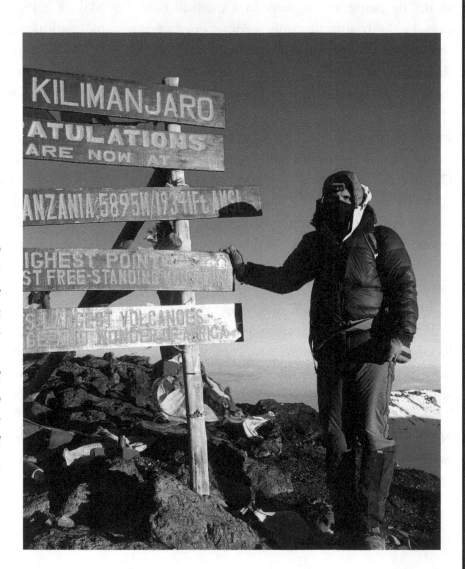

"I had to be optimistic and accept it for what it is."

Michael Rowe clocks out of his job at his family heating, ventilation, and air-conditioning business on a chilly Friday afternoon after working an eight-hour shift and immediately takes off for the Colorado mountains. The Coloradan and his climbing mates arrive late into the night to sleep before waking up between midnight and 4 a.m. They use this strategy to avoid climbing during afternoon thunderstorms in their quest to reach the summit of another 14,000-foot mountain. Michael does this thirty to forty times a year, and in December of 2017, in just his second attempt, Michael climbed the Andes' Aconcagua, which rises to 22,841 feet.

"It's truly difficult to accurately describe the sense of freedom the mountains give me," says Michael. "With little sleep and an earlier wake-up time than I have for work, most people would question why we choose to do such a thing and consider it fun. It is hard work—sometimes incredibly hard, both mentally and physically. It's also very rewarding for those five to ten minutes when you are standing on the summit in a calm wind, watching the sun rise over the horizon with a view that stretches on for hundreds of miles in any direction. Nothing else matters. It's a beautiful feeling."

Michael grew up camping, hiking, and rock climbing, and was a member of the Boy Scouts, all while coping with debilitating stomach pain. For years, his doctors attributed it to cases of food poisoning and other on-off food issues. However, at the age of seventeen, Michael's pain was so bad he was admitted to the hospital. There, he was diagnosed with pancreatitis. Each attack he got after that was worse than the one prior.

In February of 2015, Michael had an episode that trumped the others, and doctors ordered a lipase test. The pancreas makes lipase to digest fats into fatty acids. When the pancreas is damaged, these digestive enzymes can be found in the blood at higher levels than normal. Lipase results showing more than three times normal levels are likely to mean pancreatitis or damage to your pancreas. Normal is considered to be around 130 units per liter. Michael's were measured at 10,000.

His doctor immediately diagnosed him with chronic pancreatitis and ordered a blood draw and sweat test to determine if it was one of the two likeliest scenarios: cancer or cystic fibrosis. With chloride levels more than thirty points higher than the sixty needed to indicate CF, Michael was diagnosed with the disease at National Jewish Hospital in Denver in June of 2015 at twenty-three years of age.

Michael said upon being diagnosed, he dealt with the five stages of grief: denial, anger, bargaining, depression, and finally acceptance. "I had to be optimistic and accept it for what it is," he says. He began a quest to raise awareness for the disease by doing the thing he loves most: mountaineering. Over a two-year period after his diagnosis, he climbed all fifty-eight of Colorado's 14ers (mountains 14,000 feet or higher), the only known cystic fibrosis patient to do so. His journey was covered by several local news outlets, and he therefore decided he would raise money for the CF Foundation with his Aconcagua climb, asking people to donate one dollar for every thousand feet he made it up the mountain. Since that climb, he has raised just under $3,000, surpassing his goal. That number is still growing.

Michael's day, like a majority of CF warriors, is filled with enzymes, Pulmozyme®, hypertonic saline, and various antibiotics. He was actually on a two-week round of Cipro 750mg when he was on Aconcagua, taking his last dose on his summit day.

On September 7, 2018, Michael climbed to the top of Mount Kilimanjaro in Tanzania, Africa, the tallest mountain in Africa at 19,340 feet. His next conquest will be Mount Elbrus in Russia, the tallest mountain in Europe at 18,510 feet, in the summer of 2019. He also plans to climb other tall summits around the world, including completing all of the Colorado Centennial 13ers, which, including repeat trips, will give him approximately two hundred Colorado summits of over 13,000 feet.

"Unfortunately, no one can stay on the summit forever," says Michael. "We must come down, and we must clock back in on Monday. But, those beautiful moments in life, regardless of how short they may be, are what motivate me to keep climbing."

VINCENT "VINNIE" CORYELL

Age: 27   **Resides:** Colorado, United States   **Age at diagnosis:** 3 weeks

Vinnie is a world professional parkour athlete. He shares his parkour videos with his nearly ten thousand subscribers on his YouTube page. He competed in the first US-held Red Bull Art of Motion competition in 2010 and placed eighth. He went on to compete in four other Red Bull Art of Motion competitions. He has performed around the US for companies such as JEEP, Warner Brothers Interactive Entertainment, and AT&T. In 2014, Vinnie opened up the Move to Inspire Parkour Facility, which is dedicated to teaching parkour to people of all ages and abilities. Vinnie is also a founding board member of USA Parkour, the national governing body for parkour in the United States. He and his wife, Cameron, also recently opened a nonprofit Christian performing-arts company called Reverent Rhythms, which uses parkour, dance, and other art mediums to inspire and share the word of God.

"My outlook on CF has always been a positive one.
I really believe that a positive and unwavering mindset creates a healthier body."

JESSE HUYGH

Age: 28

Resides: Edegem, Antwerp, Belgium

Age at diagnosis: 12

Graduated with a bachelor of circus arts degree from Ecole Supérieure des Arts du Cirque (ESAC) in Brussels; world-touring circus acrobat who has taken part in parades, festivals, weddings, and many grand theaters

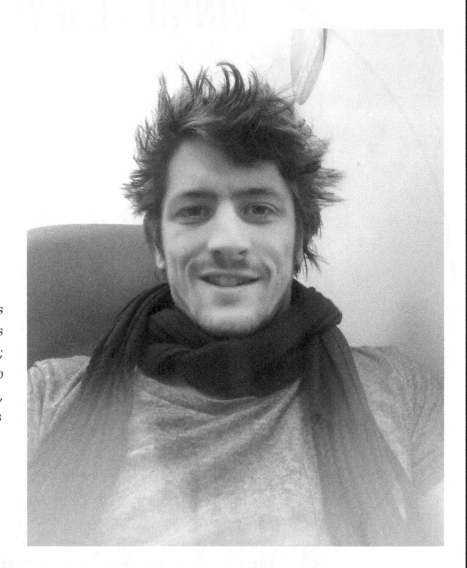

"More than anything, [CF] gave me a strength and a meaning of everyday life that lots of people seem to lose nowadays."

Jesse Huygh, a twenty-eight-year-old full-time circus acrobat, has flown across most continents performing and teaching his craft. The show must go on for this Belgium native despite a difficult journey unlike any other. It began at the age of twelve.

Despite lung, sinus, and digestive issues—he was considered asthmatic and allergic—Jesse was a very active, sportive kid. Despite the conviction of his kinesiology therapist and some of the doctors that they saw proof of CF, the diagnostics only happened when he was twelve years old. He endured sweat tests, which turned out borderline. His DNA was analyzed, which only showed one CF mutation (the Delta F508). He even went abroad to the Netherlands to see a doctor for a rectum biopsy, in which a tiny bit of Jesse's tailbone was removed so they could test the DNA in his spinal cord, before the discovery of the second mutation was finally found. This was a very rare mutation seen in less than ten other Europeans. Given the fact he had a reasonably mild form of CF, it took a long time before Jesse could finally be treated correctly.

Jesse, fortunately, was being treated for CF before he was officially diagnosed. "Luckily, my kinesiology therapist, Dirk Vandeneynde, was already treating me as such and had started teaching me the importance of autogenous drainage from the age of eight years old!" Jesse still remembers being debriefed after diagnosis as to what CF was. "That age, even though you should not be thinking of it as much as we do, you're fully capable of understanding the concepts of 'life-threatening' and 'life-reducing.'"

Following his diagnosis, Jesse was briefed by his doctor that he needed to listen to his parents and take care of himself, and that his life would be a little bit different than his peers. The real answers would come shortly after.

"My mother actually revealed to me shortly after the brief explanation from my doctor the more harsh factors of [CF]. I had some questions after listening to the doctor, so I asked her if we could talk. I came to sit next to her, and she told me that as science and the doctors these days stated, I would probably not reach an older age than twenty-five. However, when I was born, this average age would have been twelve, so science had been evolving, and without knowing we already had proven them wrong. So, we would continue doing so. My mother is still the basis of my optimistic ways."

Jesse admits that the discussion with his mother took years to digest. "Two years after, I often broke down crying in my room without understanding why. I guess it was mild depression trying to deal with this new information, this new me. But, there was so much to do—distraction, joy, love in my daily life—that it just popped up every once in a while and did not lead my ways. Hearing this from my mother made me realize the severity of the disease, the fact that I would have to up my game to fight it, face life with it. More than anything, it gave me a strength and a meaning of everyday life that lots of people seem to lose nowadays."

After his diagnosis, Jesse was followed by the CF Association of Belgium and by his local CF clinic to get the right care. It was something else entirely that he'd been doing for years that had helped keep his CF in check. Fitness was his biggest ally. He started with gymnastics as a toddler, began competing when he was about nine, and continued doing so about twenty-five hours a week until he was seventeen years old.

At fourteen years old, Jesse started taking after-school circus classes two hours a week as a hobby. The program was nonmandatory and offered two hours a week. His parents were okay with it, since it offered Jesse more chances to exercise. Soon, though, he found his passion working with the circus. The circus is not only a passion for Jesse, but his challenge, his job, and a big part of his physical and mental maintenance.

After his first full year of classes, he was asked to take part in a circus/street performers' collective in Antwerp called Ell Circo D'ell Fuego. Jesse trained in a very dusty, old castle. They had him perform in small outside events with lamp oil and fire in costumes that were washed every once in a while. "You can imagine that gives a bit more stress to a CF parent," adds Jesse, "but when the passion is there, better to accommodate it than counter it, because one will follow his passion."

When Jesse was seventeen years old, he had the opportunity to attend a circus university. He applied and was accepted to Ecole Supérieure des Arts du Cirque (ESAC) in Brussels. Seventy-eight artists auditioned that year for this highly professional physical education, and he was one of eighteen accepted. This meant a lot more to him than just being part of the university. "I don't have to tell you how that felt like a victory toward my CF. A real 'you aren't getting me down!'"

He finished this three-year education at the age of twenty and graduated with a bachelor of circus arts degree. Jesse's life has not slowed down since, as he travels all over to perform. "What I love about performing is to be exposed, transparent, and honest, and to share with the audience."

His parents helped out when they could instead of telling Jesse to stand back. "Smart move," laughs Jesse. "Joining the circus university, and thus making a clear future choice, brought them to the next level of concern, but we were in too deep already, so on we went together, me moving for my passion and life motivator, and them encouraging me and facilitating my ways."

Now he was doing up to forty hours of repetitions per week on top of the two he already did, and performances in all sorts of stuff. He took part in parades, festivals, weddings, and many grand theaters. From age fourteen on, the circus pretty much took up his life.

He credits a lot of his success to his family. "They have helped me face my fears and make those fears my strengths." Jesse lost his mom to heart-and-vein issues when he was twenty-one. He said his father has spent the most time in the hospital, not as a patient, but as the one visiting Jesse's mom and Jesse whenever he was hospitalized.

CF still plays a role in his performances. "It is limiting me in cardiac endurance, and therefore has an influence on how I rhythm my performances, how I keep pushing those limits, and how I grow to have a better understanding of the necessary physical phrasing (movements) as it goes on."

As far as taking care of himself, he travels most of the year, but still is home every few months to visit his doctor. If he feels poorly on the road, he is able to Skype with her to see if he needs to change his medications or add an antibiotic. Jesse is very regimented and does nebulizers in the morning and at night, takes enzymes with meals, and carries an emergency box with antibiotics, cortisone, and a contact number for the local CF organization and kinesiologist in the region where he is performing.

His dream is to continue with his awesome profession. He says it's all about "continuing performing and growing to be a better artist and person."

For Jesse, the show must go on.

BEN MUDGE

Age: 29

Resides: Belfast, Northern Ireland, United Kingdom

Age at diagnosis: 3 days

Graced the cover of Men's Fitness UK; *has won multiple physique/bodybuilding championships; briefly worked as an assistant director on* Game of Thrones; Men's Fitness *Trainer of the Year 2016*

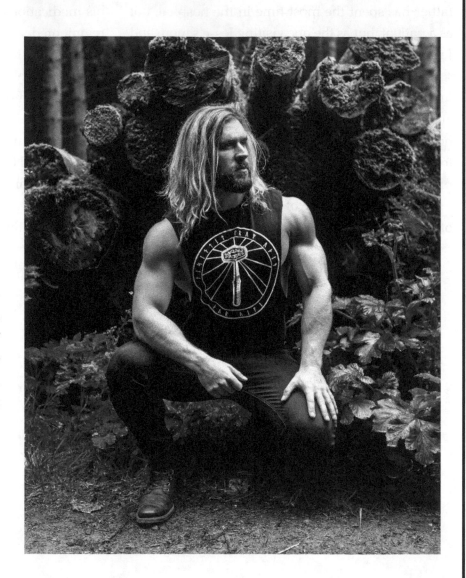

"I realize more and more how fortunate I am to be doing as well as I am, but a big part of this is all the work that I put in."

If you venture out to a gym in Belfast, Northern Ireland, and spot a 5'9", 190-pound chiseled male with long blond locks, sixteen-inch biceps, and a forty-five-inch chest, blink and you might think that you just saw Thor. Ben Mudge is proud of his resemblance to the fictitious superhero, but Ben's been a superhero in his own way.

Ben was three days old when he was diagnosed with CF, but says he never felt different from anyone else while growing up. "My parents did a great job of that," he says, "and for that, I cannot thank them enough." Ben says his CF issues growing up were mostly digestive, as he was hospitalized twice for bowel obstructions.

True awareness of the disease didn't occur to him until leaving secondary school. "I was on the small side, but I wasn't the smallest," says Ben. "It was upon leaving school, thus leaving the strict regime of organized sports like basketball, rugby, and track and field, that I noticed my health drop a bit. I then decided to go to the gym with my friends at age sixteen and really enjoyed it. I then started to focus on my career, which was in the film-and-TV industry. I wanted to be a director."

Ben says that leaving school at sixteen was not unusual in Northern Ireland, as students have a choice to go to school for another two years to complete their A-levels, or go out into the workforce. He says that he was the only one amongst his friends who left, because he did not do well in a standard school environment.

The Belfast native boasts an impressive public résumé that includes being on the cover of *Men's Fitness UK*, a six-page feature in *Muscle & Fitness*, winning physique/bodybuilding shows, and even working briefly as an assistant director on *Game of Thrones*.

"The long hours and lack of sleep and exercise were proving to be very difficult for me," he says about his time on *Game of Thrones*, in which he had to look after the cast as well as the show's extras. "It landed me in the hospital for the first time with a chest infection." It was then that Ben decided he needed to change his career into something that would allow him to be active and healthy, and he now says building a successful business as a personal trainer is his proudest accomplishment. "In this capacity," he says, "I can also work directly with children with CF and encourage them to take their medicines and just to be more active."

Ben, who is still often confused for Thor because of his long blond hair and impressive physique, knows that kids look at him as a superhero. While he considers that an honor, he knows that image gives him a lot of responsibility.

Ben says his personal goals are driven by the fear of the consequences of CF, which keeps him working hard in the gym. "As I get older," he says, "birthdays have taken on a different meaning for me. I realize more and more how fortunate I am to be doing as well as I am, but a big part of this is all the work that I put in. I hope I can help children realize their best adult life starts now!"

JES DAVIS

Age: 29

Resides: New York, United States

Age at diagnosis: 3

Debuted her own line of leather jackets at New York Fashion Week in February 2017; star of many off-Broadway plays; seasoned actor of film, theater, and TV including roles in Netflix TV series Orange Is the New Black, The Punisher, *and* Russian Doll

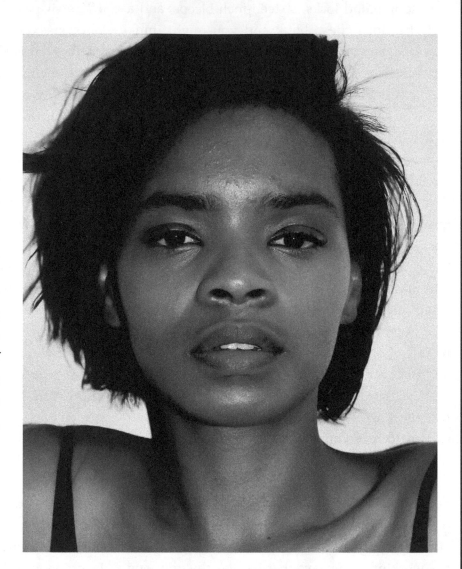

"CF has taught me so much about perseverance, which is an experience that I may not have had otherwise."

"That's not something that black children have," the doctors told Jes Davis' mother when she pushed for a CF test for Jes and her little brother, Jason, who is two years younger. Only one in fifteen to twenty thousand African American births account for someone born with CF, so it was up to Jes' mom to prove that she not only accounted for one of those births, but two.

"Thankfully, Mom observed foods our bodies couldn't process—including soy and non-fatty foods—and tailored our diets even before getting diagnosed and given the proper meds."

Jes' mother has a medical/science background and was able to deduce from Jes' abdominal issues that something was wrong. "I don't remember if there was much coughing, but there was a lot of constipation. I was just constantly in pain for the first three years of my life. But, what really tipped my mom off about my brother was the smell of his bowel, and he was also having horrible constipation. She would have to massage his tummy to help him move his bowels. She told me that during a doctor's visit for the two of us, as she was changing my one-year-old brother's diaper, the nurse expressed surprise at the smell and confirmed for Mom what she already knew—'That's not normal.' And, that is what got us tested. Prior to that, the doctors we had visited accused her of making us sick, which was a whole other challenge for my mother."

After the positive diagnosis, Jes and her brother were equipped with the proper meds and treatments. However, despite their mom's education, acute observational skills, and determination, it became clear that a comprehensive treatment plan and even strict adherence to that plan could only do so much.

"I was in and out of school from getting lung infections, viruses," says Jes. "I would go to the bathroom a lot during class because I had a small bladder, and I weighed only forty-nine pounds in the fifth grade, and the assumption by my peers was that I was bulimic [or] anorexic, for which I was taunted.

"I hated the idea of being weak, and CF, to me, for a long time, was a permanent weakness that I would forever have. Now, not so much. Everyone has stuff they deal with, and no one is better or worse for it. My brother and I were told that we wouldn't make it to sixteen. I'm twenty-nine. My brother is twenty-seven. Maybe those living without chronic illness don't have to cope with death in that way so early on in life. When you're a child, you are granted invincibility. Your parents don't talk about death. They don't tell you right off that life is not infinite. We had to learn and accept that early."

When Jes got to high school, she was exhausted with the badgering. Not only was she not bulimic or anorexic, as her classmates taunted, she was actively trying to *keep on* weight! Jason, meanwhile, was having his own issues. He was out of school with lung infections and viruses.

"He also wasn't socializing that well and

preferred to be home," says Jes. "So, my mom made the executive decision to have him homeschooled. I followed because I was exhausted, but more so I just didn't really care for my peers and preferred to be alone. I hung out with friends outside of school, but I didn't have many people in school I needed to be around. CF did and didn't influence this. A part of me feels that even if I didn't have CF, I probably would have liked to be homeschooled."

On top of CF, Jes and Jason have both been diagnosed with clinical depression. "He takes meds for anxiety. I opted for talk therapy and more natural remedies to manage my mood," says Jes. "As a kid, coping with CF and depression went hand in hand. Most of what my depression was about was the fact that I had something that other kids didn't have, that I was not only different because of my personality, but also because of my insides—my body was fighting me. I decided to keep a journal and write down all my thoughts concerning CF and my depression to understand where they crossed paths, which was helpful."

Growing up, Jes coped with her conditions by focusing on her art. "Creating is therapeutic," says Jes. "Someone who is sick can't create, I thought, which is stupid, but I thought this because it was helpful to distance myself sometimes, and at the same time, a detriment. I've come to a place where I can accept being someone with a chronic condition and be a creator."

Jason initially tried to escape his mental demons by getting lost in books and video games before he, too, found solace in artistic expression, his choice mediums being stand-up comedy and writing. Jes' calling was the dramatic arts. "Acting is great because I can disappear into another person/character and not have to consider life as a CF patient," she says, "but as someone who doesn't have to do treatments and take meds or cough."

Jes' passion for live theater led to parts in many off-Broadway plays, her most notable being *Northbound*, in which she played a young slave woman who is in an abusive, incestuous relationship with her half-brother, the slave master's son. Her acting talents translate to screen, as well, as she has a small, recurring role on the hit Netflix series *Orange Is the New Black*.

As Jes has refined her acting craft, she has found her way back to a greater appreciation for the arts in general. "I live in the art world!" she says, and proves her devotion through her writing, singing, painting, and designing. She started her own design brand called TUNC, which features custom, punk leather jackets she debuted at her first fashion show in November 2016. In February 2017, she debuted a new jacket line at New York Fashion Week.

"CF was my enemy for a while because I didn't understand it, and because I didn't understand it, I fought it. I treated it as the bad part of myself, and because there is no cure, it was the bad part of myself that would always be there. My overall perception has changed. CF has taught me so much about perseverance, which is an experience that I may not have had otherwise. I no longer see it as trying to kill me, because it's essentially a parasite. It needs me to survive. Otherwise, it dies. We have to work together to keep this body working. It's actually like my sidekick, in a way, and not really my enemy anymore. My work now is about understanding it. Being healthy is the ultimate goal."

BIANCA NICHOLAS

Age: 30

Resides: London, England, United Kingdom

Age at diagnosis: 2

Founded the Cystic Fibrosis Virtual Choir in 2017, a group of CF singers who perform "virtually" so as not to risk bacterial cross-contamination, which was featured on the Christmas Top 40 Charity Album "Stand Together" in the UK that same year

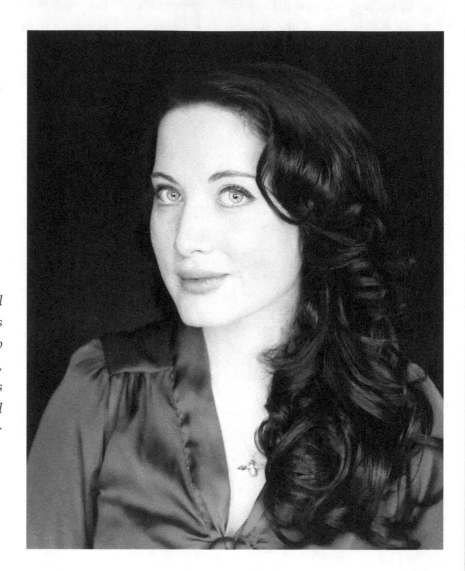

"It's wonderful that the thing I love more than anything in the world helps me manage my condition so well."

When Beckenham, Kent–born Bianca Nicholas was thirteen, her nurse, Peggy, at her initial visit at the CF clinic at Lewisham, asked the petite, brown-haired, blue-eyed girl if she'd ever been granted a wish, and what would hers be. Bianca didn't hesitate. "I knew straightaway that mine would be something to do with singing." Neither Bianca nor her nurse could ever imagine where that dream would lead her.

Bianca was born in 1989, the same year the CF gene was discovered. As a baby, Bianca would cry a lot, especially after she ate. Her family noticed that though she ate a lot, she was not putting on weight, and then came the other famous symptom: she had extremely salty skin. She was eventually diagnosed with cystic fibrosis at the age of two.

Growing up, Bianca's parents were very supportive, but made sure that she took very good care of herself. "They pushed me to pursue everything I was good at and did not allow it to ever feel like CF was something that could hold me back."

Bianca's career into show business took off early when, at nine years old, she starred in the short film . . . *Is It the Design on the Wrapper?*, which won the Palme d'Or award at the Cannes Film Festival. Then, at eleven, she landed a small role in the movie *Sleepy Hollow* alongside movie legend Johnny Depp.

Bianca says her mom would do postural drainage to loosen the mucus in her lungs, a therapy that Bianca now performs on herself. She learned early on from her parents not to be ashamed of her disease and to be open about it. Therefore, she says that she was not fazed by the disease as a youngster. "I guess I didn't realize that not everyone had it. It was only when I became a teenager that I began to realize that I was different from my peers and became a little more self-conscious about it."

Bianca admits that it was difficult being open regarding some things having to do with CF. When she was eleven, she first read about the median life expectancy for people with CF online. "This was not a conversation my parents had with me, and I felt like I'd been hit by a train. I shook the feeling off very quickly. I told no one. I didn't want to upset anyone. So, I just tried to be brave and forget about it."

Bianca always had dreams of a musical career. Hers started when, at fifteen, she was granted a wish by Starlight Children's Foundation, a national charity that grants wishes for terminally ill children and provides entertainment in hospitals and hospices.

A few years later in 2008, she auditioned for *The X Factor*. In 2009, while her singing career was just taking flight, so too did her personal life. She met a gentleman named Gearoid while on a holiday trip at an Irish bar in Majorca, Spain. "It was love at first sight," says Bianca. While Bianca was still living in England and Gearoid was living in Ireland, the two continued their long-distance relationship. About this time, her first single, "Hold On To Your Dreams," was launched in 2011, entering the Top

100 singles chart and reaching number one on the iTunes vocal chart. In 2014, she would appear on *The Voice UK*. She has also toured and performed for both Princes William and Harry.

While all of this was going on, CF was along for the ride, too, though perhaps Bianca tried to ignore it. In 2014, that mindset had to change. "In 2014, I developed pseudomonas for the first time in years. I had become a bit lazy with my treatments, and it was a real kick in the butt to show me CF is still with me and a serious condition, and I needed to start taking it seriously again."

While Bianca, who also needs insulin and regular blood testing due to being diagnosed with CF-related diabetes, refocused on her CF by being compliant with all of her therapies, she also admits that singing has been a big contributor to keeping her lungs as healthy as they are. "It's wonderful that the thing I love more than anything in the world helps me manage my condition so well."

In 2015, she performed as part of a duet with Alex Larke called Electro Velvet singing "Still In Love With You" in front of two hundred million people in the Eurovision Song Contest on the BBC. She and Alex were chosen from hundreds of contestants to perform. To support her and raise awareness and funds to research a cure, the CF Trust encouraged people to take a selfie holding their breath, share it on social media with the hashtag #breathe4bianca, and also donate funds to the CF Trust.

Following all of her singing success, Bianca had nine hospital stays in six months and numerous courses of IV antibiotics, as well as a bout of sepsis due to an infected stent in her kidney. Those times were tough, but she was able to get better and return to the stage.

In 2016, she and Gearoid were finally married. The following year, Bianca recorded two cover tracks in the world-famous Studio Two at Abbey Road, which also hosted recording greats such as the Beatles, Pink Floyd, and Adele.

Bianca understands that she is a role model to others with CF, but she does not want to be judged based simply on having the disease. "I really don't want to be defined by [CF]. It's so important to be an individual away from the illness. I don't want to be the girl with CF who sings. I want to be the singer who happens to have CF."

TRAVIS FLORES

Age: 28   **Resides:** California, United States   **Age at diagnosis:** 4 months

Travis Flores, a two-time double-lung-transplant survivor, wrote The Spider Who Never Gave Up *in 1999 at the age of eight. The book was published in 2004, just short of his thirteenth birthday, to provide hope for hospitalized children. Disney printed the book in 2005 and raised over $1 million. Travis went on to make a speech that brought in a remarkable $2 million in one night for the Make-A-Wish Foundation® on June 18, 2005. Mayor Michael Mullen of Marietta, Ohio, a city near Travis's hometown of Newport, Ohio, proclaimed June 18 to be henceforth known in Marietta as "Travis Flores Day."*

"We must not question the things we do not understand.'Allow them to unfold, and they will be answered in the time they're meant to be."

JONNY SIMPSON

Age: 31

Resides: Cumbria, England, United Kingdom

Age at diagnosis: 6 weeks

Personal trainer, fitness model, and brand ambassador; 2012 and 2013 Mr. Elite bodybuilding champion; competed in the finals of Top Model® 2018 in the UK

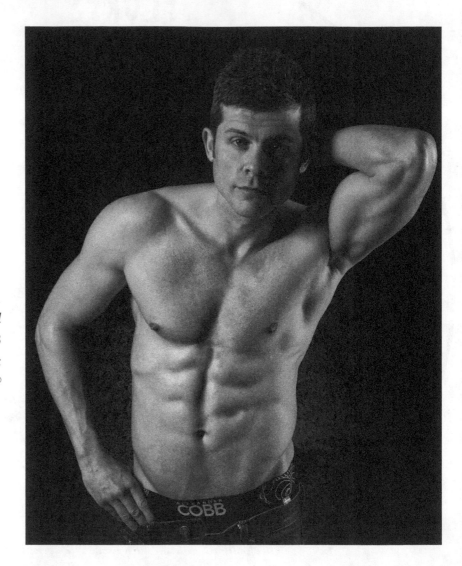

"I have been very lucky to have shared my accolades all over the world, but the most important accomplishment is being able to live a normal, active life."

Jonny Simpson's seemingly unlikely story of bodybuilding success began six weeks into his life, when he was diagnosed with CF. "I was very sick growing up," he says, "and my body never fully developed because of this, spending a lot of my youth in the hospital."

Dealt all sorts of ominous statistics by health professionals about the devastating consequences to life expectancy, fertility, and other items too big to be processed by a teenager, Jonny felt resigned to a life sat peering out of the same hospital windows. It was as if the world had left him behind.

That all changed a few months before Jonny's nineteenth birthday. "I remember the day I beat my depression," says the 2012 and 2013 Mr. Elite bodybuilding champ, "and that was October 10, 2005. It was one of the most liberating days of my life, and my CF has never controlled or defined my future ever since."

For a long time as a teenager, Jonny felt isolated and like his chances were bleak of living a normal life. "I decided I needed to make some serious and drastic changes. I am not sure what the exact catalyst was for me deciding enough was enough. Maybe I had exhausted myself on being a victim of circumstance. It finally sunk in that only I could change the outcome. Nobody could do it for me. That notion can be very empowering if you have the right perspective."

It was at the age of nineteen that Jonny took the bull by the horns. Understanding that medication can only do so much, "I decided to start focusing on my fitness and nutrition," he says. By combining it with a healthy lifestyle, Jonny seemed to be on to something.

"I started forcing myself to eat and doing whatever exercise I could. I remember trying to stop myself from throwing up from the amount of food I was eating, and coughing up a lot of blood when I began training hard. Looking back, these symptoms were unnecessary, but I was so desperate for change.

"When I began, I struggled to walk up stairs and couldn't squat a bar with any weight on it. People used to laugh, but that soon all changed when I stuck at it. Every improvement I made, I reminded myself of where I was going and took a picture of the day I started training, reminding myself that if I stop, then that picture is what I would go back to. I still use it as my motivation today, but discipline is the most important factor.

"I was sick of feeling so low, having zero energy, and despising the person I saw in the mirror, not just from an aesthetic viewpoint, but from who I had allowed myself to become. I went to some pretty dark places in those years.

"I had some old five-kilogram dumbbells that I had bought from a friend when we were still in school. They were very light, but I never used them, so for years they just collected dust. I started using them every day.

"I wasn't very clued up on what to do at first, I

just started eating as much as I could and lifting the light weights that I had. I tried doing body-weight exercises also—literally anything I could do at the time, I tried.

"As I improved, I began to buy more equipment to train at home. Then, after I had built myself up a little, I joined a gym, and I've never looked back since! I became healthily obsessed with the gym and how I could make my body change. I wanted to learn as much as possible, and am still learning today. I entered my first bodybuilding competition, which was aired on primetime TV, launched my website, and everything just took off from there. I landed sponsors and a lot of publicity. It was very cool to see all of my hard work pay off."

Jonny managed to gain seventy pounds (ninety pounds to one hundred sixty pounds) over eight years and remain at the same body-fat percentage, adding a miraculous 35 percent to his FEV1. This then led Jonny to share his story in the media and online, seeking to connect with other people with CF and try to encourage them to do the same. Jonny says that since 2010, he has been using social media to help others. "It's always an amazing feeling to get to share my story with the world. It's something I have tried to do as much as possible, so I appreciate and seize every opportunity that comes my way."

Jonny's passions extend beyond and even enhance his successful career as a model, bodybuilder, and face of Fight Life, an international brand of supplements. "I love anything creative—literature, music, and cuisine, to name but a few," he says. "I have been very lucky to have shared my accolades all over the world, but the most important accomplishment is being able to live a normal, active life. I feel like I am living my life now, something I didn't do for the first eighteen years."

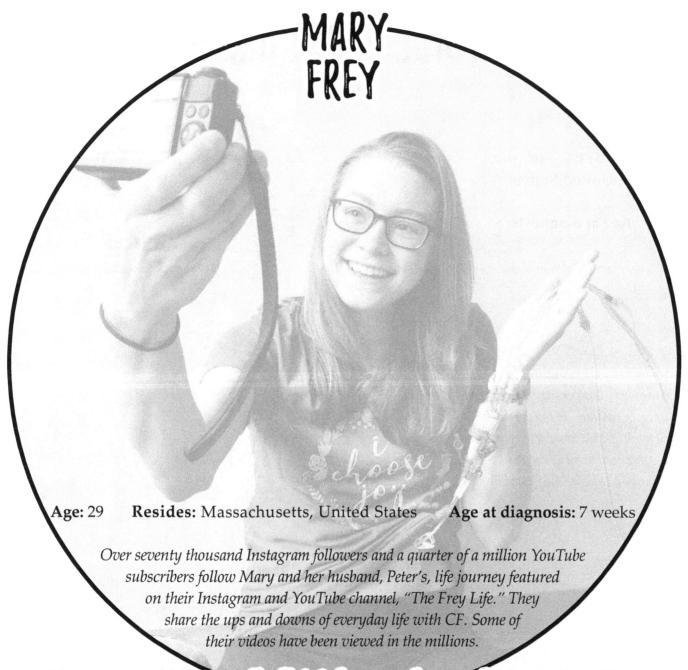

MARY FREY

Age: 29   **Resides:** Massachusetts, United States   **Age at diagnosis:** 7 weeks

Over seventy thousand Instagram followers and a quarter of a million YouTube subscribers follow Mary and her husband, Peter's, life journey featured on their Instagram and YouTube channel, "The Frey Life." They share the ups and downs of everyday life with CF. Some of their videos have been viewed in the millions.

"Health doesn't necessarily dictate how my day, week, or month will be. I have a choice to choose joy amidst the hard work, the coughing, and the pain!"

BILL ELDER JR.

Age: 31

Resides: California, United States

Age at diagnosis: 8

Stanford University undergraduate; graduate of the Boonshoft School of Medicine; currently doing his residency at the Santa Rosa Family Medicine Residency

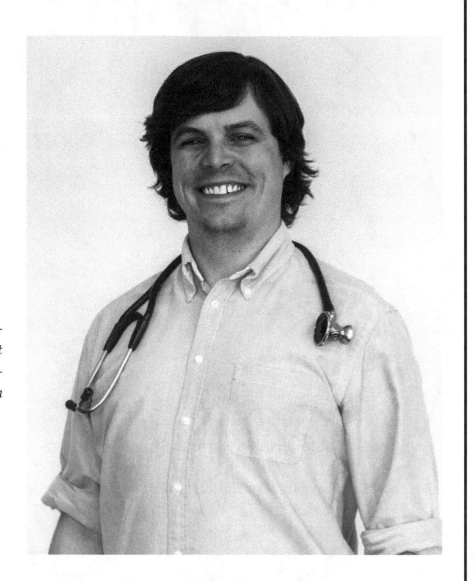

"I spent a lot of time thinking about how I could have a positive impact on the world with the time I have."

Bill Elder Jr. truly means it when he says that cystic fibrosis changed his life for the better. The diagnosis at eight years old not only helped to alleviate his symptoms, but also took him on a career path to change the lives of others.

Bill was raised in the Rocky Mountains of Colorado. In retrospect, running and playing at 7,648 feet above sea level likely helped his lungs become stronger and healthier.

Bill's symptoms came to light when he began having recurrent debilitating abdominal pain around eight years old. Bill saw many specialists and was given numerous working diagnoses, from lactose intolerance to Crohn's disease. A more comprehensive approach might have revealed that clubbed fingers had been noted in a prior emergency department (ED) visit. After numerous doctors' appointments, he was referred to the gastroenterology clinic at Children's Hospital Colorado. A sweat chloride test confirmed CF.

"As strange as it sounds," says Bill, "I was thrilled to be diagnosed with CF. Suddenly, I had enzymes that I could take before meals to prevent abdominal pain, and I was able to live my life again. Although I was only eight years old, Dr. Frank Accurso took the time to answer my seemingly endless questions, eventually drawing the CFTR chloride channel on a whiteboard and teaching me the underlying pathophysiology of my disease. It was not the medications, but the time my doctor spent speaking with me that changed my life."

Bill's mom, Teresa, remembers that time, as well. "Dr. Accurso asked Bill to tell him what medicines he was taking and why. I started to jump in and help answer, and Dr. Accurso gently stopped me, and Bill answered in complete detail. It was a good learning tool for me, too. Dr. Accurso always made time to answer our parent questions after he exhausted Bill's long list of science-related questions. Bill was clearly meant to be a doctor."

From that day on, Bill knew that he wanted to learn everything he could about CF and use his newfound passion for medicine to one day improve the lives of others. "This passion led me to volunteer in my community and work on CF research in high school. My parents, my younger brother, Andy, and I became involved with the CF Foundation. We first worked with the Colorado Rockies and then did Great Strides, bike rides, galas, and any other activity that could get us closer to a cure. I became comfortable talking about CF to adults and large groups."

From fourth grade through ninth grade, Bill's family moved frequently, from Colorado to the San Francisco Bay Area to Florida to Los Angeles, all for his mother's career. It was during this time that he had his first epiphany about his life expectancy. "When I was about thirteen," he says, "I started to realize that the life expectancy of those with CF was, at that time, in the late twenties or early thirties."

Bill remembers bringing the issue up to his mom. "Our family had always been into racing, and my dad had just gotten his dream car, a Porsche 911 C4S, after racing Alfa Romeos for years. I asked how old my dad was now that he had gotten his dream car, and my mom said he was in his forties. I replied, 'Oh, so I won't live long enough to get my dream car.' She was pretty taken aback and discussed that we have no idea how long my life expectancy will actually be because there are so many new medications on the horizon."

Bill embraced his mother's assertion and hitched optimism on the scientific possibilities of a cure for CF. Then, as he was starting high school, Bill's family moved back to Colorado, reuniting him with Dr. Accurso and the team at the Mike McMorris Cystic Fibrosis Research and Care Center at Children's Hospital Colorado. "Dr. Accurso, a great teacher as well as CF researcher and doctor, let me intern with him and work on a CF research project. He taught me statistics and the thrill of discovering new knowledge."

Bill began to learn a lot about the disease and applied his newfound knowledge to his own health. "In high school I was still needing frequent tune-ups with IV antibiotics, but the more I learned about the pathophysiology of CF, the more devoted I became to my treatment regimen. Using the vest daily with all of my nebulizers took a lot of time, but always felt like an investment to keep me out of the hospital. Running was also a huge part of staying healthy for me. I learned that while running, another ion channel in the lungs (the ENaC, epithelial sodium channel) is inhibited, which keeps more salt in the mucus (and therefore more water). Thus, when I was running, my lungs were more similar to normal lungs and my mucus was thinner."

Throughout high school and college, Bill fell in love with evidence-based medicine and would critically appraise any new CF articles that were published. At the time, he did not realize that the skills he was developing in the areas of comprehensive care, evidenced-based medicine, and public service would align so naturally with family medicine.

"When I was in high school, I thought there was a good chance I could live to be about forty years old, and I spent a lot of time thinking about how I could have a positive impact on the world with the time I have. This calling was solidified at Stanford University when I volunteered at the Bridge Peer Counseling Center. Being able to be there for my peers in their moments of crises was humbling and made me realize that I could serve others by pursuing medicine."

While at Stanford, he dove headfirst into science courses from nearly every discipline. "I was drawn to the ideals of humanism, respecting human agency, and using rationality to address societal needs," says Bill. "As my study of philosophy continued, I began to delve into ethics and distributive justice, which transformed my desire to help others into a personal calling to serve those around me."

His faith was tested, as he recalls one of his sickliest CF moments occurring at the end of his freshman year. "Living in the dorm, with the constant circulation of viruses and studying or staying up with friends until the wee hours each night, had worn me down over the year," says Bill. "I remember feeling completely exhausted and beat down as I went into my CF appointment at the start of summer. After many tries with my best effort, I found that my FEV1 had decreased by over a liter of air. I was crestfallen.

"Thankfully my family, friends, and CF care team rallied around me and encouraged me to fight back. I went in for a tune-up, adding another scar to my left arm from the PICC line, and started going for long daily runs in between all the IV antibiotics, nebulized medications, and therapy-vest sessions. I regained almost all of my lost lung function that summer."

Then, Kalydeco came along, and Bill remembers to the minute when his faith in medicine was validated. "I would often look at the CFF drug pipeline and take hope from the progress and the many people who have helped get us to this point," he says. "Then, on February 15, 2012, at 8:30 p.m., I took my first dose of ivacaftor (Kalydeco). At 3:30 a.m., I realized I was able to breathe easily in and out of my nose, which I hadn't been able to do in decades. I sat on the floor making notes for about forty-five minutes, trying to convince the scientist in me that this was real. I was able to breathe, deeply filling my lungs and sinuses, including my small airways. My sense of smell returned.

"When I realized this truly was a profound change, I ran down the hall, pounded on my parents' bedroom door, and exclaimed, 'Kalydeco is working! Kalydeco is working!' We sat there in the dark, my parents in tears, as I described my ability to breathe and smell. In the following days and weeks, my health continued to improve. I was able to run for longer distances, even in the thin air of Colorado. My FEV1 improved and I gained a healthy fifteen pounds."

After graduating from Stanford and the Wright State University Boonshoft School of Medicine in Dayton, Ohio, Bill matched into the Santa Rosa Family Medicine Residency and advocated for the CF community locally and nationally. In 2015, he was a guest of First Lady Michelle Obama during the State of the Union address. It was at this event that President Obama mentioned cystic fibrosis as a prime example of how nonprofits, the pharmaceutical industry, researchers, patients, and their families can work together to produce more targeted and effective treatments in precision medicine.

Now as a resident in Santa Rosa, California, who will finish his residency in July of 2019 and become a board-certified family physician, Bill is able to use the insights gained from being a CF patient to provide empathetic and evidence-based care for his local community.

EMMAH EVANS

Age: 31

Resides: Adelaide, South Australia, Australia

Age at diagnosis: Birth

Wife; mother of two; former National Youth Ambassador for Cystic Fibrosis Australia; Cure4CF Foundation Australia ambassador; model; author and international empowerment speaker; writes a popular blog called CF Mummy

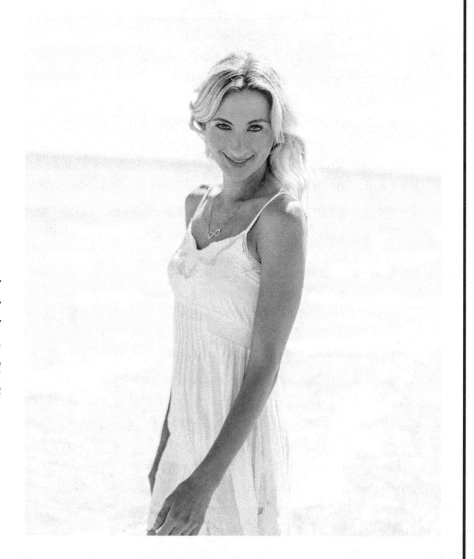

"Disability, visible or invisible, is no reason to fail."

Joy and Arnie Money both wanted a child very badly, but not just any child. Arnie was a paraplegic who participated in power weightlifting in the Paralympic Games in Seoul, Korea, in 1988, and he and Joy specifically wanted a child with special needs. Around the same time that he was competing, a young girl was born and immediately diagnosed with cystic fibrosis. Her birth parents were told the newborn Australian would not survive and decided to give her up. Joy and Arnie jumped at the opportunity to add this baby, Emmah, to their lives.

Emmah says she is grateful to have her adopted parents in her life because they are so supportive of her. Her early days were not easy; she spent much of her childhood fighting lung infections. One year, she spent a total of sixteen weeks in the hospital. Things only got worse as a teenager. "My CF declined. I struggled with depression, anxiety, and the loss of several childhood friends to cystic fibrosis."

In the beginning of her final years of school, Emmah became ill and was not getting any better. She was spending more and more time in the hospital to fight infections. To make matters worse, she was being bullied because she was always sick and missing school. Cyberbullies were the main culprits, often sending texts with the acronym RIP.

Things started looking up for Emmah, though. After months of intravenous antibiotics, her health suddenly improved, and she was even granted a wish from the Make-A-Wish Foundation at the age of fifteen: a three-week trip to Australia's Gold Coast, the family's first holiday together. There, she got her wish to model a surf-wear line and keep all the clothes. This also opened a lot of doors for Emmah in the modeling profession.

Following that, she attended a new high school where, in 2005, she won a national Australian girls' magazine competition for *Girlfriend* magazine thanks to her positive impact in the community, which included creating and attending CF fundraisers, as well as campaigning for Australians with CF to have access to the drug Pulmozyme, eventually leading to government approval. This turned out to be Emmah's first encounter with fundraising and advocacy. Emmah took the $3,000 prize money and donated it back to Cystic Fibrosis Australia for their Cure4CF campaign. To date, Emmah has raised more than $50,000 for CF Australia. Soon after the magazine hit newsstands, she began traveling and talking of her experiences with CF, leading to her becoming the National Youth Ambassador for Cystic Fibrosis Australia.

"I was fortunate to travel around Australia at numerous fundraisers, galas, corporations, and schools where I could share my story and motivate others."

Emmah released her autobiography, *The Words Inside*, in 2006, in which she speaks openly about being adopted and her battle with cystic fibrosis.

Emmah and her husband of three years, Nick,

who have been together a grand total of thirteen years, were able to have two children. Their daughter, Ayvah, six, and son, Logan, four, were conceived naturally, and while both are carriers, neither has cystic fibrosis.

Emmah's thoughts on being a mom are that it's a bit more challenging, but she wouldn't change it for the world. "They get germs and bugs, so I catch them naturally, but then I seem to get knocked more than anyone for a longer period of time. This is my full-time job. My day genuinely consists of the morning treatment routine, from inhaled treatments to finding 'normal' ways to do physio, like the gym or a beach run [or] walk. I repeat this sometimes in the afternoon, but definitely at night, so twice a day I am doing intensive hours of treatment to keep my health at a 'good' level." Emmah also takes enzymes with meals, as she is pancreatic deficient.

Emmah, who jumps out of airplanes and goes shark-cage diving for the sole purpose of raising awareness for cystic fibrosis, is now the ambassador for the Cure4CF Foundation, an Adelaide research team that she is confident will find a cure for CF in the years ahead. Emmah also spent three years campaigning for Orkambi to be government-subsidized, which has recently been approved in Australia for cystic fibrosis patients. She writes a popular blog about her life as both a CF patient and a mother of two called *CF Mummy*, and is now working on a second book. She does not do as much modeling these days, though she did do a runway show on Mother's Day of 2017. She still goes around giving speeches and attempts to be an active role model for the CF community in order "to inspire, motivate, and give hope to all that disability, visible or invisible, is no reason to fail."

A lesson she no doubt learned early on from her father.

ALI CHRISTENSEN WILDE

CHRISTINA CHRISTENSEN STUTZMAN

Age: 29

Resides: Colorado, United States

Age at diagnosis: Birth

Age: 23

Resides: Utah, United States

Age at diagnosis: Birth

America's Got Talent *Top 10 finalists in 2010*

Sisters Ali and Christina Christensen became famous in 2010 for reaching the Top 10 on America's Got Talent, a hit TV show on NBC. The night their audition aired, the Cystic Fibrosis Foundation website crashed because so many people were looking up CF. The two sisters went on a twenty-four-city tour after the show to continue sharing their message. They have performed at many CF fundraisers and have helped raise millions of dollars toward cystic fibrosis research.

"Our parents taught us that we were not different.
They taught us that we could do anything we put our minds to." (Ali Wilde)

VERÔNICA STASIAK BEDNARCZUK

Age: 32

Resides: Curitiba, Paraná, Brazil

Age at diagnosis: 23

Mother; wife; blogger; psychologist; first patient to become a member of the Brazilian Cystic Fibrosis Study Group; founder and director of Instituto Unidos pela Vida (United for Life–Brazilian Institute for Cystic Fibrosis Care)

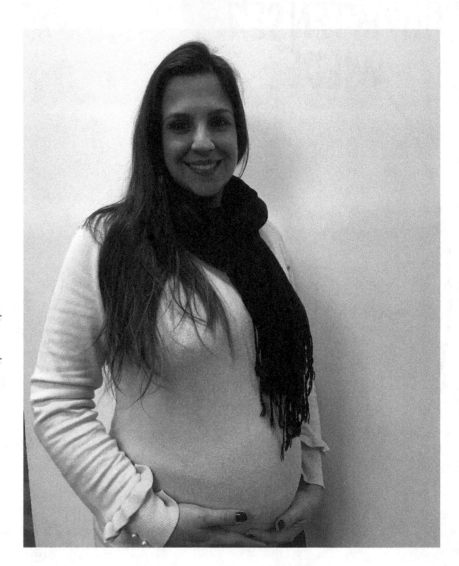

"When I finally got my diagnosis, I was scared, but I tried to look at it as a gift, a chance to live longer and better."

Verônica is a psychologist and founder and director of Instituto Unidos pela Vida (United for Life–Brazilian Institute for Cystic Fibrosis Care). She herself got involved because, at the age of twenty-three in September of 2009, she was diagnosed with cystic fibrosis.

Verônica always had serious health problems. She had roughly five pneumonias per year since she was a child, had multiple surgeries to remove two pieces of her right lung, and another procedure to remove her gallbladder. Only after a severe battle with pancreatitis did she finally get the diagnosis of cystic fibrosis. Her doctor never suspected the disease because CF was not very well known in Brazil, and Verônica had a family history of asthma. Immediately after her diagnosis, she switched to a CF specialist.

Verônica has studied CF extensively since her diagnosis, and she realizes that all the serious health complications she had throughout her life arose from the lack of early diagnosis and appropriate treatment. Therefore, she decided to help people who could be in the same situation. First, she began a blog, which explained cystic fibrosis and discussed her life, and after a year, she founded the Instituto Unidos pela Vida. Today, the institute is the largest Brazilian nonprofit organization developing projects related to cystic fibrosis.

"We offer support to all people seeking help with us—parents at the moment of diagnosis, people with CF, and health professionals. We also have around three hundred volunteers around Brazil helping us to disseminate CF in their communities. Representing the institute, I'm part of the committee organizing the National Congress of Cystic Fibrosis, the most important event about CF in Brazil."

While Verônica increased national awareness in the nine-plus years since her diagnosis, Brazil is still quite far behind other countries like the US in terms of public policy. Thus, the largest institute is actually quite small. Along with two dedicated assistants, Verônica is responsible for everything to keep the organization working, from the fundraising up until the project development and management. She also gives lectures at companies, hospitals, and universities as a strategy to disseminate CF.

"I wish," Verônica continues, "in ten years, all patients in Brazil could get their diagnoses as soon as possible, they could know their genetic mutations (unfortunately, the majority of patients in Brazil still don't know), and could access the newest medications and therapies." Verônica has dreams for herself, as well. "I also hope in ten years, my own CF would be increasingly controlled." She has obvious incentive thanks to the event that occurred on December 11, 2018. She and her husband of five years, Vinicius, welcomed their first child, Helena. "She was conceived naturally and all is going well," says the exuberant mother.

"[Having a child] was mine and my husband's dream, and with much love and care, it [has been] fulfilled!"

ASHLEY BALLOU-BONNEMA

Age: 32

Resides: South Dakota, United States

Age at diagnosis: 1 month

Author of the memoir Breathing Bravely: Giving Voice to CF; *writes a blog called* Breathe Bravely; *started an organization called* sINgSPIRE; *local and national advocate for the CF Foundation and those fighting cystic fibrosis*

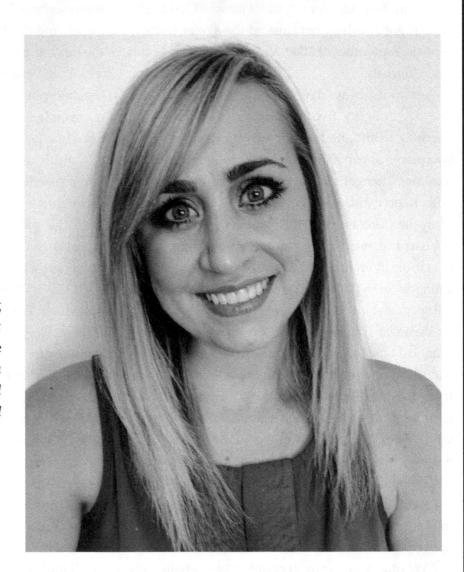

"I was an ordinary kid growing up in an unusual world of circumstance."

Cystic fibrosis singer—rarely are these three words connected. But, in the case of South Dakota's own Ashley Ballou-Bonnema, there is no better way to describe her.

Ashley used to stand in front of her family's TV dancing and singing along to MTV music videos. Her dad, Steve, would tape the videos so she could watch on repeat. As she got older, she would put on mini concerts in her childhood-home basement, "Complete with track lighting," jokes Ashley. "Throughout my childhood, I always loved singing my heart and lungs out."

To Ashley, singing was the escape she needed from the stranglehold cystic fibrosis put on her family.

Ashley was born the second of two children with CF. Her brother, Nate, was seven years older than her and was not diagnosed until he was six years old, only after a long and rigorous search for answers. She knew from a very young age that she and her brother shared the same disease, but they seemingly lived very different lives. His life was spent within the walls of a hospital, while every night she got to leave those walls and return to the bed in their childhood home.

"I was an ordinary kid growing up in an unusual world of circumstance. My early childhood was not spent climbing the monkey bars or racing down slides. It was spent with a huge extended family of nurses, respiratory therapists, and doctors amongst the jungle gym of IV poles and the cold tile of sterile hospital rooms. My life revolved around 'living' at the hospital with my brother, me being most frequently a visitor. Our house just seemed like a place in which we used to merely sleep, store our car for the evening, and where the school bus would pick me up. My brother would maybe come home for a week—most of the time on home IVs—and then proceed to spend weeks in the hospital. During my own inpatient admissions, Nate would be across or down the hall on the same PEDS floor, and my parents would hop from room to room throughout the days and nights."

That was, until Nate finally lost the battle to cystic fibrosis when Ashley was ten.

Ashley, and of course her parents, were devastated. Ashley said Nate's death eventually led to her parents' divorce. While Ashley was obviously distraught, she did not see his CF as the same as hers. "Growing up, I never thought of myself as sick. That could be in part to constantly watching my brother live the definition of 'sick.' From a young age I remember taking enzymes, but I didn't begin nebulized treatments or CPT until early elementary school. During those elementary years, I don't remember frequently coughing or ever feeling like I couldn't breathe, even amidst a childhood cold."

Following Nate's death, Ashley's mom, Linda, bought her a piano, and she began taking music lessons. "That really propelled my love for singing and music." Ashley also admits singing helped her lungs and also provided mental and emotional stability.

"Through middle school and teen years I remember 'feeling my lungs' for the first time, and my delayed growth and maturation became glaringly evident in comparison to my peers. I still have those same 'chicken legs' and birdlike arms my adolescence made me so conscious of."

While Ashley didn't see her CF as the same as Nate's, the disease still frightened her. "For as long as I can remember, CF has been very real. It's been something I've feared. It's been something I've watched firsthand mercilessly steal the life of someone I loved."

Her fear caused her to try to conceal her CF from the world. "I saw how the disease hurt the people I loved, and I didn't want to be cause to their pain." For years after Nate's death, Ashley tried putting many of those memories and experiences of the past at arm's distance. However, feelings of survivor's guilt would follow her for the rest of her life.

Concealing CF became a theme that would follow Ashley from middle school, to high school, and even college. A part of her believed if she could keep it hidden from people, then it clearly didn't exist. But, CF did exist, and it wasn't going anywhere.

Ashley eventually relied on her passion for singing to help her move forward. It was in high school that her best friend, who often heard Ashley sing in choir, told her that she needed to try out for the school musical. "I remember that moment because for the first time I felt that my love for singing was justified and that it was made even better because I could share that love with others."

Ashley performed in musicals, choir, and took a few lessons here and there during junior high and high school. As a senior in high school, she began taking formal lessons at the local university thirty miles away.

She ended up going to a small private college where she graduated with a bachelor of art in vocal music and French. During college she had the great opportunity to sing as a part of a prestigious choir, traveling through Europe on incredible tours and domestically across the United States. There were a few speed bumps along the way with CF that called for rounds of IV antibiotics, but mostly, no one knew she had CF, not even her closest professors. In fact, one of Ashley's greatest accomplishments was fighting her way back from a devastating exacerbation and a lung function of 25 percent to six months later standing on a stage giving her graduate-degree voice recital with 54 percent lung function.

After college, she spent some time in Germany studying opera and doing extensive travel. Again, she thought she was invincible and did everything she could to hide her CF. But, there were things about CF that were becoming more and more difficult to conceal, like infections, hospitalizations, the reality that the medications that were used had lost their potency to her CF, and progressive complications she simply could not control. So, during her first year of graduate studies, she made the choice to be open and honest about her life with CF. On April 1, 2014, Ashley finally let the cat out of the bag.

"I started a blog called *Breathe Bravely* that shared my honest life with CF. I never would have imagined the response it got and continues to get. It is something that is still beyond words for me to describe." The blog has been published on the *Huffington Post* more than thirty times and is now a nonprofit organization that has published its first book, *Breathing Bravely: Giving Voice to Cystic Fibrosis*, which shares Ashley's journey with cystic fibrosis.

In addition, her organization is launching several programs specific to giving voice to CF, including one that marries her love for singing with combatting CF called sINgSPIRE, a ten-week program that combats cystic fibrosis through the art of singing. Individuals with CF are paired with professional voice instructors and take private voice lessons via video calls for ten weeks following their specific sINgSPIRE program. Through the art of singing, sINgSPIRE promotes self-awareness, increased respiratory strength, good posture, and most of all, expansive and thoughtful breathing. The art of singing and Ashley's program not only result in physical betterment of breath management and overall respiratory awareness in those with CF, but also psychological betterment through increased endorphins, increased perceived breath management, and decreased anxiety.

Following completion of her graduate program in vocal performance, she built a private voice studio of twenty-five students. Ashley continues to sing for special events with different organizations and ensembles.

Ashley, now in her early thirties, is married to her high school sweetheart, Mark. They live in Sioux Falls, South Dakota, with their two dogs. She continues to follow her passion for singing while defying the expectations placed upon her by CF by taking her diagnosis and turning it into a meaningful direction: empowering others with CF to know the positive impact singing can have on their own lives and, as Ashley puts it, how to "find the beauty in every breath."

SABRINA WALKER

Age: 32

Resides: California, United States

Age at diagnosis: 4

Wife; mother; non-Hodgkin's lymphoma survivor; finisher of about a dozen half marathons; 2017 Chicago Marathon finisher; 2018 New York City Marathon finisher

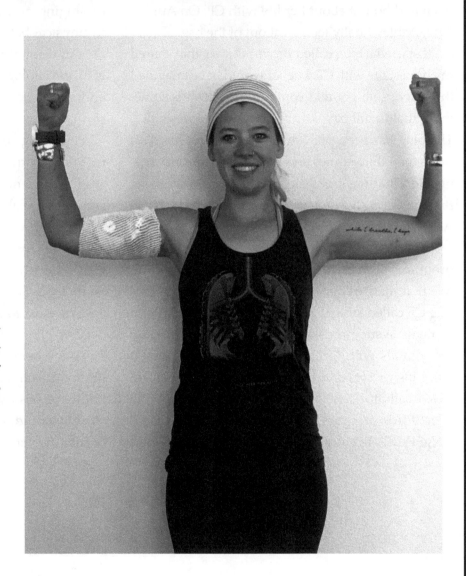

"Cystic fibrosis and cancer are not excuses to keep me from running. They will continue to fuel the fire that inspires me to run."

When young Sabrina Smith, an Alaska native of the Tlingit tribe, was diagnosed with cystic fibrosis, doctors told her family that she wouldn't live past the age of eight. After blasting past that milestone thanks to new treatments, she began using running as a vehicle to live longer.

She began training at twelve years old. Her father, a physical-education teacher, thought the activity would be healthy for her. Sabrina's mom supported the idea and regularly took her to a track to help instill the importance of a routine.

"My main motivation for running has been to outrun cystic fibrosis and to prevent further lung deterioration," says Sabrina. "Exercise is a part of what keeps me healthy. It is a part of my airway clearance, and helps me rid the mucus out of my lungs. I am determined to run and exercise for my health."

As Sabrina moved through her teens, she seemed to be on top of her health . . . until disaster struck during her senior year of high school while running cross-country. She started to feel random back pain, her right foot began going numb, and she lost weight rapidly. After doing an x-ray of her spine, her doctor found a tumor. She was officially diagnosed with non-Hodgkin's lymphoma in 2005 at the age of eighteen.

Sabrina was angry, wondering why someone with a terminal disease had to also deal with cancer. She admits to feeling a little depressed, but knew the only thing she could do was be positive. Three weeks later, she began chemotherapy.

All told, she did four months of chemotherapy and one month of radiation before finally being declared to be in remission. Sabrina has now been in remission for nearly fourteen years.

After surviving another health scare in 2011 when her lung function reached an all-time low, Sabrina returned to her former passion: running. Though the return to running was not easy, she was dedicated to keeping herself in the best possible shape. Shortly after, she saw on Facebook that Team Boomer (a program from the Boomer Esiason Foundation that encourages people with cystic fibrosis to incorporate fitness in their lives) was doing their inaugural four-mile Run to Breathe at Central Park in New York City, and decided that she should celebrate her health and her upcoming college graduation by running in it.

Sabrina and her long-term boyfriend, Adam, trained for months before jumping on a plane to New York. After participating in Run to Breathe, Adam asked Sabrina to be his wife. "It was one of the greatest days of my life," she says.

Adam and Sabrina had been married for three years when they decided to talk about having children. "It was something that we knew could be an issue, but we never really talked about it until after we were married," says Adam. Adam was tested and did not have the CF gene, and being that Sabrina was declared healthy enough by her doctors, they gave it a go. Sabrina was pregnant soon after. Other than experiencing gestational diabetes, Sabrina had a noneventful pregnancy as she and Adam welcomed their son, Leo, into the world.

After Leo was born, Sabrina continued to stay in shape and train, sometimes pushing Leo's stroller while running in the snow. She once again ran for Team Boomer while raising funds, then she signed up for the Chicago Marathon in 2016. "I trained for four to five months. My runs varied from three to ten miles, and my long runs went up to eighteen. I was running four to five days and averaging forty miles per week." Sabrina not only completed the marathon that year, but completed the New York City Marathon with Adam the following year. It's not difficult to understand her reason for running and staying in good health.

"I have a child and husband who need me," says Sabrina. "I want Leo to grow up with his mom. I want to be able to teach him to be kind, humble, to follow his dreams, strive for greatness, learn from failure, travel, read, be respectful, gain knowledge through experience, and pick himself up when life is tough. Leo is my inspiration to lace up my shoes and get out there and run."

While Leo inspires Sabrina, it's Sabrina who inspires Adam. "She is absolutely the strongest person I know," he says.

Today, Sabrina's weekly exercise routine varies, but usually consists of group exercise classes, hiking, and of course, running. She clocks twenty to thirty miles a week and has run about a dozen half marathons. "Cystic fibrosis and cancer are not excuses to keep me from running. They will continue to fuel the fire that inspires me to run. Running is a way to keep my soul, lungs, and body happy. I have the ability to run, and I will continue to do so until it is not possible. Running keeps me alive!"

MARKÉTA MIKŠÍKOVÁ

Age: 30   **Resides:** Prague, Czech Republic   **Age at diagnosis:** 3

Markéta works as the fundraising and public-relations manager for the Cystic Fibrosis Foundation in the Czech Republic. She organized an annual calendar with photographs of a dozen Czech women with cystic fibrosis called "Salty Women" to raise money and expand knowledge about the disease. In three years, approximately three thousand calendars have been sold, which has raised approximately $50,000. She's also writing a CF book about Czech patients, due out winter of 2020, called Life with Salty Taste.

"If you cannot find a way for yourself, try to start helping other people, and it will help you more than you expected."

ANDREA GOLDMAN

Age: 34

Resides: Florida, United States

Age at diagnosis: 6

Wife; mother; post-transplant lymphoproliferative disorder (PTLD) cancer and double-lung-transplant survivor; half-marathon finisher

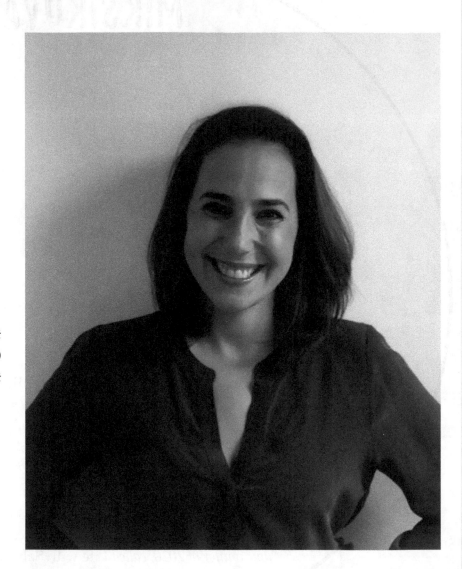

"I knew I was going to wake up. I knew I was going to get my life back."

After retiring as a guidance counselor and going on disability, Andrea's symptoms stabilized enough for her and her husband, Adam, to reopen the conversation about having children. They had talked about the subject in the past, but Andrea hesitated because she didn't know how much time she had left. Adam told her to look at it another way: "You have so much to give and such a great heart. This baby would be brought into the world with love."

Andrea grew up in South Florida. However, due to the fact that there were not any true CF specialists in her area at the time, she ventured to the University of North Carolina (UNC) Children's Hospital and later the University of Cincinnati Children's Hospital for her CF clinic appointments. She chose these centers based on the clinics' and doctors' reputations.

Andrea says that growing up, her mom, JoAnn, would put CF into perspective by saying, "You like to dance, your favorite color is purple, and you have CF. It is part of you, not all of you."

While she says her symptoms were "mild" growing up—she was hospitalized three times before the age of eighteen. They got tougher as she got older, which led to more hospitalizations. One tune-up stands out. "It was my senior year of high school and my Grandma Bea, with whom I was extremely close, came to see me in the hospital," says Andrea, who lived only fifteen minutes from her grandmother and would spend almost every other weekend at her house. Grandma Bea taught Andrea how to swim, came to her school plays, and attended almost all of her dance recitals. Andrea calls her mischievous, "but in a fun way! She had advanced lung cancer, and told me that we would both beat this."

This buoyed Andrea, but two months later, in October of 2002, Grandma Bea passed away rather suddenly, her departure leaving Andrea grief-stricken and, for the first time, hit with the realization that she herself had a real terminal illness. "I always thought when someone passed away from an illness, the family is somehow prepared. They are sick, the doctors let you know there is nothing more you can do, you say what you need to say, and that's how you get closure. That wasn't it at all. My grandma went into the hospital with GI pain and I never saw her again. How could she die without me knowing it was coming? [Would] that happen to me? I felt totally lied to about how people lose their battles with disease. It got me thinking about my own death and how I would be able to give closure to my loved ones."

She soon found a therapist and, through trial and error, was prescribed the proper antianxiety meds. Andrea learned that she could not predict the future and had to be positive.

Following her grandmother's passing, Andrea was hospitalized at least twice a year, had her gallbladder removed, and even contracted the Epstein-Barr virus, which led to a two-week bout of mono. Lung exacerbations became even more unpredictable from age twenty-three on.

In July of 2012, she'd been dating Adam for nearly three years. He says that faced with making a decision to spend the rest of his life with someone with a terminal illness, he knew one thing for sure: "I absolutely loved an incredibly special and unique person, and could not imagine living without her. For me, eventually, those feelings overrode all of the worries that had consumed my mind since I met [Andrea]."

He surprised Andrea by taking her out on a sailboat and proposing to her that evening. All of their closest family and friends were there. "I was living on cloud nine," Andrea gushed.

The following Monday, she visited her doctor for a regular appointment. The doctor and nurse coordinator came into the room with serious looks and said it was time to consider a transplant due to Andrea's recently low PFT of 29 percent. Andrea felt defeated, confused, and that her life was over, and this after just getting engaged to Adam.

Andrea did not have the strength to call Adam after she received the news. It wasn't until she returned from the doctor and Adam came home from work that she finally told him. His head hung low and he was speechless. His eyes grew watery. Andrea decided to throw herself into wedding planning so she could take her mind off of things. Despite her low lung function, she was not feeling miserable health-wise at the time, so a transplant was not imminent.

Andrea and Adam married in March of 2013. During the wedding weekend and honeymoon, she was suffering with undiagnosed CFRD and fevers. Once diagnosed, things got better, but it seemed like every happy moment came with a more difficult one.

In September of 2013, they started the IVF process, and by August 2014, after three attempts, their surrogate was pregnant. Andrea still remembers receiving the news. "My honest reaction to the good news was panicked. I called Adam hoping his excitement would help snap me out of it. I felt confused. My health hadn't been that great. I had just gotten back from a hospital stay. I started Googling the due date wondering where I'd be health-wise. I felt isolated and guilty because I knew I was going to need new lungs soon. Yet another example of how even with a long-awaited pregnancy, CF changed how I got to experience it."

Andrea's symptoms worsened again and she was on oxygen 24/7 beginning in December 2014. Finally, in January the following year, she was told she definitely needed a transplant. "I remember bringing my oxygen tank to Zumba and yoga classes prior to my transplant," says Andrea. "I used to dance competitively, and it was humbling to struggle through the classes so much." Still, Andrea found comfort taking the classes, as the women there were very encouraging.

The day after her thirtieth birthday in March of 2015, they relocated to Durham, North Carolina, for a double-lung transplant at Duke University. At this point, Adam and Andrea's child was due in just a month and Andrea was pent up with anxiety, wanting more than anything to be there when the baby was born. Her lung function was around 20 percent at that point, and she needed the transplant soon. The doctors told her she would be too sick to travel to see the birth of her son, so they came up with a different plan. Once the baby was born, he would be brought to Durham to live with her. Adam, her mom, and her mother-in-law would be there to help.

On April 24, Andrea was doing laps around the track as part of her rehab when she was summoned over the loudspeaker to head to the conference room. Andrea and Adam's surrogate had gone into labor in Orlando. Adam was in Orlando and called Andrea so she see could witness their son's birth on FaceTime. Bryce's birthdate had already been predetermined due to Andrea's surrogate having high blood pressure issues around the thirty-seven-week mark.

"It was a mixed blessing, as I wanted Bryce to be born when he was ready, but at the same time, now we could plan the logistics around his arrival."

Adam, his parents, and Andrea's brother, father, and sister-in-law drove to Orlando to be there when Bryce was born. Andrea's best friend and cousin, Missy, along with Missy's mom and Andrea's aunt, Linda, arrived in Durham to help make the birth as exciting as possible for Andrea, as they understood how difficult it was for her to not be there. Andrea said after the hour spent "virtually" with her son, it was time to disconnect. She experienced a great deal of sadness that she could not be there for the birth in person.

Adam, on the other hand, was dealing in his own way. "The only way to deal with the simultaneous impending birth of my son in Orlando and double-lung transplant for my wife in Durham was to compartmentalize and focus on the here and now. Fortunately, and likely out of necessity, compartmentalizing and taking things day by day had become somewhat natural for me by this time. So, although it was heartbreaking not to have my wife with me while our son was born, I was able to focus all of my energy on the birth of my son."

Bryce was born on a Friday, and the hospital in Orlando did their best to get him checked out and ready to meet Andrea. He was off with Adam and his parents to Durham by that Sunday morning.

"It was surreal to meet Bryce," says Andrea. "It was a little uncomfortable because there were so many people around and someone was videotaping our first meeting. But, once I had our first moment alone and we touched skin to skin, it started to feel real."

Now it was time to focus on her own health. While being evaluated for her transplant, Andrea said the one thing she wanted to do to celebrate her new lungs was to do some long-distance running. First, of course, she had to get new lungs.

After two false alarms, Andrea was finally rolled into the operating room on May 23, 2015, just twelve days after being listed for her double-lung transplant. "I was very excited when the lungs were a go. I made all of my phone calls to let everyone know the good news. I never thought this was something to be afraid of. I knew I was going to wake up. I knew I was going to get my life back."

She said goodbye to an emotional Adam, and although she wanted to, she could not say goodbye to Bryce. He was sleeping when she received the call, and babies were not allowed in the pre-op area when it was time to have the surgery.

While all of this was going on, her cousin, Missy, a lactation consultant and nutritionist, was able to network between friends and family to find more than twenty women to donate six months' worth of breast milk to Andrea—an amazing amount of breast milk. Missy raised money to pay for these women to ship the frozen milk overnight.

Andrea started walking miraculously within twenty-four hours of her transplant. "[Bryce] was my motivation to wake up and start walking and moving as soon as they took the breathing tube out. I was away from him for nine days and I didn't want to miss anything. I remembered the doctors telling me that to get out I had to be able to walk one mile around the floor for seven days straight, so that was in the back of my mind. When I started walking, it felt like I was running a marathon. The nurses were cheering, clapping, and showing all sorts of encouragement on either side of me."

Amazingly, only eight days after surgery, she was discharged. Things were finally looking up. As soon as she moved back home a few months later, she was taking workout classes with other moms who didn't know Andrea prior to her transplant, so they had no idea the battle that she had fought. "For all they knew, I was just a person trying to get back into shape."

In October, five months following the transplant and now living in Boca Raton, Andrea developed a fever that lasted four weeks and led to several misdiagnoses. X-rays eventually revealed several tumors, and Andrea was diagnosed with post-transplant lymphoproliferative disorder (PTLD). The cancer was caused by the drugs she took to suppress her immune system after the transplant, but that were at the same time reactivating the Epstein-Barr virus she contracted at the age of eighteen.

"When I found out I had cancer, I was in pure shock," says Andrea. "I thought my transplant was going to be the hardest thing. It never seems to end."

She endured six rounds of five-day, twenty-four-hour-a-day chemo over the course of four months that included New Year's Eve and Day, Valentine's Day, her wedding anniversary, and her thirty-first birthday. "It was crushing," says Andrea, "because we talked about how we would celebrate each of these occasions once I received new lungs, and undergoing cancer treatment was certainly not part of any of the celebration plans." Adam and Bryce once again inspired her to endure the physical and psychological challenges.

"In the end, one of the only guarantees in life is its unpredictability," says Adam. "In light of the incredible medical miracles and technological advancements that occur seemingly every day, and all of the other unknowns that await every one of us in our life's journey, I made the decision to spend my life with the woman I loved, grab all the happiness I could along the way, and to look forward to being surprised. Despite watching my wife endure the most unimaginable of circumstances, I can honestly say I made the best decision of my life."

Andrea was declared to be in remission after the four months of chemo. Finally able to celebrate good health, she followed through with her goal prior to her transplant to do some long-distance running.

She, along with two other women with CF, one of whom had a transplant just six months after Andrea, decided to train together to run the Disney Princess Half Marathon in Orlando, Florida. Andrea knew the training would be difficult, but for once it was Andrea in control and not her disease. "When you're sick with CF, you have to push through the pain of surgeries at no choice of your own, but this time it was my decision to put myself through pain."

Andrea endured the six months of training and the thirteen-mile trek on February 25, 2018, to complete the half marathon—and in turn, complete her comeback story.

While Andrea has had a number of different challenges over the last few years, she admits that her motivation has never wavered.

"This whole journey has been for Bryce."

XAN NOWAKOWSKI

Age: 35

Resides: Florida, United States

Age at diagnosis: 32

Assistant professor in the Geriatrics & Behavioral Sciences and Social Medicine departments at the Florida State University College of Medicine; evaluator for the Florida Asthma Program; serves as the evaluator for the Geriatrics Workforce Enhancement Program; founded Write Where It Hurts, an advocacy project for scholars doing trauma-informed research

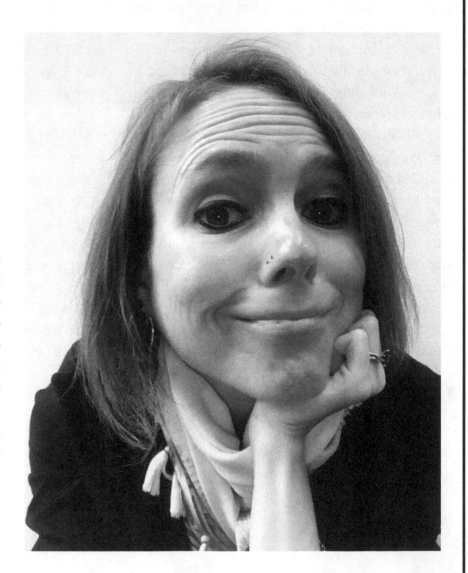

"Like many others with CF, I am tough, resilient, and incredibly stubborn, and I am fiercely determined to live a long life in service to others with CF!"

"Getting diagnosed and finally being able to access coordinated CF care has changed my life in wonderful ways," says Xan Nowakowski, a medical sociologist and public-health program evaluator who studies patterns and disparities in how people age with complex chronic conditions. "I developed a strong interest in health research, probably as a result of growing up in neuroscience labs and clinical classrooms at a medical school."

From birth, Xan suffered from distal intestinal obstruction syndrome (DIOS), thick mucus like rubber cement, chronic bronchitis and pneumonia, reactive airways, poor digestion, steatorrhea, arthritis, recurrent sinusitis, and upper respiratory infections.

Xan's childhood doctor was a lung specialist, and was always convinced that they (Xan is agender and therefore asks to be referred to as "they") had CF. "He treated me as best he could, and my lung function stabilized for a while with the kind of care that was standard in the late eighties and early nineties."

Xan's battle against undiagnosed cystic fibrosis was not without its triumphs. "My care was basically a trial-and-error process of seeing which drugs would help me and which ones would hurt me," says Xan. "I began using some supplements to help me get food energy, plus vitamins and minerals. I learned to avoid foods that made my chronic diarrhea worse, but remained baffled about why I would sometimes get obstructions. It seemed

contradictory that I would need to manage both issues at once, unless I really did have CF."

Despite having a few successes, Xan's health declined throughout their teens and twenties, and they developed a variety of complications. "I got a somewhat incoherent hodgepodge of pulmonary-care services from an allergist who was pretty sure I had CF. He was the one who ordered the sweat test when I was five, but I did not find out until much later that the test was done improperly. The care staff conducting the test could barely get any sweat off my skin, as I have a low resting body temperature and rarely sweat. But, even the small sample they got contained a high amount of chloride."

It wasn't just a dearth of CF services in New Jersey in the 1980s and improper care coordination that delayed the diagnosis and prolonged the complications. "There was the additional problem of people not listening to me or my family," Xan says. "My parents knew what was happening, but they could not prove it because they were not medical doctors. It became a terrible catch-22, with doctors thinking I would surely have been diagnosed already if CF were responsible for my myriad issues."

Then, on the night of May 24, 2007, at twenty-three years old, Xan was admitted to the cardiac intensive-care unit at Robert Wood Johnson University Hospital in Hamilton, New Jersey. Xan's heart had become so damaged because of complications from CF—which would not be fully diagnosed for another nine years—that they wound up with long QT syndrome (a type of arrhythmia). The attending physician in the emergency room had never seen a serum potassium level that low on a living human being, and thought it unlikely that Xan would survive the night. Xan had other ideas, though. "As a nurse placed an IV in my arm and hooked me up to a heart monitor, I looked at the doctor and said, 'The hell I'm dying. Fix me!'

"The next few days were difficult in a variety of ways, but I survived," says Xan, "and the experience taught me much about the importance of caring for people as complete beings rather than mere clusters of pathologies. I began working on my admissions essay for my public-health graduate program in the patient lounge on the telemetry ward, and those days became the start of a tremendously purposive career in health-services research."

Still undiagnosed, Xan earned a master's in public health (MPH) in one and a half years while working full time. They built a great career with that degree, quickly returned to school, and finished a master's of science (MS) and PhD in medical sociology in exactly two years and ten days. "A few weeks shy of my thirtieth birthday—a birthday my doctors thought at one point that I would not live to see—I got hooded at my doctoral graduation ceremony," Xan says. "That moment where my parents slipped the hood over my head and hugged me in front of the entire university administration was one of the most affirming of my life.

"At age thirty-two, my lung function had come back up a little, but I showed up at my doctor's office with a vasculitis rash and a nasty infection that had spread throughout my urinary system and kidneys. My doctor sent me to a hematologist and also sent over six years' worth of bloodwork reports and medical records. Literally the first question the specialist asked me was whether I had ever been tested for cystic fibrosis. From that initial meeting with me and the physical exam he did, he was ninety-nine percent sure that I should have been diagnosed with CF as a child. This was confirmed when a couple of months later I moved to Orlando and was able to connect with much more experienced CF specialists."

Xan had finally received a positive cystic fibrosis diagnosis. "I face a lot of challenges, both physically and emotionally, because of how long I went without a conclusive diagnosis or appropriately comprehensive care. I still experience all of the anger, fear, and disappointment that goes along with living with so much catastrophic damage to my body at age thirty-five as a result of not being listened to when I was younger. But, despite having bronchiectasis, I still have my original lungs and can blow an FEV1 score in the high nineties when not dealing with an active infection. Like many others with CF, I am tough, resilient, and incredibly stubborn, and I am fiercely determined to live a long life in service to others with CF!"

ANDY SIMMONS
(A.K.A. "ANDY BOY SIMMONZ")

Age: 34   **Resides:** Hampshire, England, United Kingdom   **Age at diagnosis:** 13

Andy has wrestled in the Frontier Wrestling Alliance (FWA), the Wrestling Alliance, International Pro Wrestling: UK, 1 Pro Wrestling, Real Quality Wrestling, World Wrestling Entertainment (WWE), Irish Whip Wrestling, and Revolution Pro. He debuted on WWE RAW on October 15, 2007, and was even introduced by the legendary Vince McMahon. He currently runs one of the most successful wrestling schools in the UK, Revolution Pro Wrestling, and teaches classes four times a week.

"It's all about the power of positivity!"

HANNAH CAMIC

Age: 35

Resides: Pennsylvania, United States

Age at diagnosis: Birth

Graduated high school as both class president and class valedictorian; mother; marathon runner; teacher of chemistry and forensic science; raised more than $72,000 for the Cystic Fibrosis Foundation as a member of the Run to Cure CF team

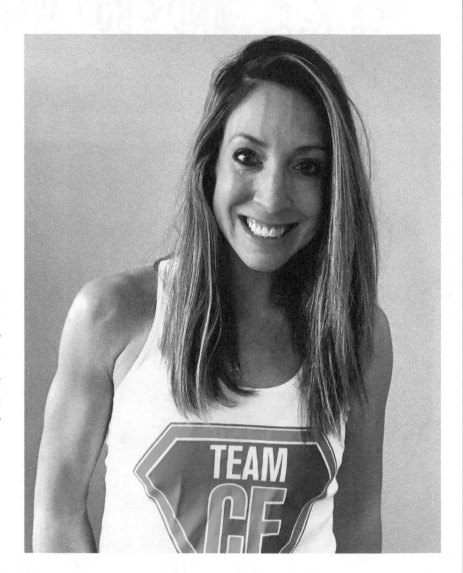

"I feel you miss out on a ton in life if you allow your fear of failure to stop you from experiencing all the amazing opportunities this world has to offer."

"I received meconium ileus surgery and spent the first couple months of my life in the hospital," says Hannah Camic, who did not let her difficult debut prevent her from making a difference. The thirty-five-year-old Pennsylvanian is entering her sixth year as a member of the Run to Cure CF team as part of the Dick's Sporting Goods Pittsburgh Marathon, a platform that has helped her raise more than $72,000 for the Cystic Fibrosis Foundation. "Despite the battle beginning from day one when I was diagnosed with CF, I was always a fighter and belong to a strong, loving family of fighters. I am the middle child and only daughter. I have an older brother, Jake, who also has CF. [He] and my brother Levi, who does not have CF, have always done their best to take care of [me] and pushed me to achieve all my dreams with a no-excuse attitude."

Hannah says that despite her and Jake having CF, the focus of the family was not on the disease. "Growing up, my parents loved us all equally, supported us in every way possible, and made sure we took full advantage of life. They made sure we were as healthy as possible, and we followed a strict treatment regimen, yet CF was not the focus of our lives."

While CF wasn't the focus of her childhood, Hannah remembers one day at age eleven when it played an integral role. Hannah, who kept her condition to herself so that she would be treated like everyone else, recalls sifting through the mail and picking up a newsletter that came from the doctor's office. "I read that the average life expectancy was in the twenties," she says, "I was shocked—horrified! I always just thought I had to take pills and do breathing treatments. Sure, I got sick a little more often than my friends, but I was not aware of what it really meant to have cystic fibrosis."

While the news was unnerving, Hannah didn't let it prevent her from living her life. She attended Bucknell University on a full scholarship, where she majored in chemistry and received her teaching certificate. It was during her college days that she had her first PICC line. She moved back to Pittsburgh, got married, and began her teaching career.

Hannah turned her attention to running in her late twenties. "I haven't always been a runner. What started as a slow mile has turned into running nearly four thousand miles and eighty races ranging from a mile to a marathon to relays. Running has served as a form of physical therapy for me, as the pounding on the pavement helps to loosen the thick mucus clogging my airways and makes me feel like I have a victory over cystic fibrosis."

The races themselves as a member of the Run to Cure CF team, well, that's a different story. Hannah recalls the happenings during the first three years specifically. Year one, Hannah was scheduled to compete in a half marathon. "My training and fundraising went extremely well . . . until the week before. I came down with quite the cold, but still had my heart set on completing the race. Instead, I found myself watching the race on local TV with IVs and tubes hanging out of my body. I was devastated.

"I was released [from the hospital] late on Sunday, [and] the next morning I decided that my mourning time was over and that I needed to complete the race. I went online and found out Cleveland's half marathon was in two weeks. I called my family who lived out there, and my cousin already had the mindset I did. We would run the race together. So, two weeks later, with perfect weather and the support of my amazing family, my cousin and I crossed the finish line in less time than I imagined. As they placed the medal around my neck, I couldn't have imagined a better feeling."

Year two as part of the fundraising team, Hannah managed to run a full marathon despite the fact that she probably should've been in the hospital. "Training went amazingly well," she says. "I surpassed my fundraising goal, and all was good until the week before the race. I got sick—really sick. I spent about five hours a day desperately trying to clear my lungs so that I could finish the race, or at least start it. Knowing I wouldn't come close to achieving my goal time, I insisted on running the race. I finished in over five hours, heartbroken that my time did not match up with my training. I ended up with a PICC line a few weeks later. That was not the best way to kick off my summer."

The third year competing to raise money for the CF Foundation, she ran two marathons in May following 24/7 IVs *and* a twenty-mile training run with an IV pump in her backpack. She admits she did not reveal this stunt to her family, as she knows they would not have been thrilled with her choice, but she deemed the completion of the two marathons and the training run a success.

Hannah knows her efforts may seem "a bit insane," but there's a method to the madness. "Some people may think I'm a glutton for punishment," she says. "Why would I subject myself to all that training, with the possibility of a repeat of the past? Well, I feel you miss out on a ton in life if you allow your fear of failure to stop you from experiencing all the amazing opportunities this world has to offer."

Hannah's running milestones are quite impressive, but she also maintains a full-time job as a teacher of chemistry and forensic science at Bethel Park High School in Pittsburgh, Pennsylvania, takes care of her family, and is proud of how her running exploits have helped raise funds for the CF community. And, while Hannah loves to run, that's not her biggest motivator. "My number-one motivation has dark, curly hair, a heart-melting grin, and goes by the name of Noelle. She is my nine-year-old daughter and the greatest motivator you could find. She gives me the strength to complete my three hours of treatments each day and take the best care of myself I possibly can."

In 2017, Hannah ran her fastest marathon to date at 4:25:59 and crossed the finish line while holding Noelle's hand.

"Despite staying positive, CF brings some tough times. On the difficult days, I draw strength from the hope of being around to raise Noelle. I long to hear about her first love and witness her graduate high school. That is why I refuse to give up. I want to be there for all the smiles and wipe away the tears. I dream of the day when we run our first race together."

For Hannah, that's the most important race of all.

NATALIE CRAWFORD

Age: 36

Resides: Northampton, England, United Kingdom

Age at diagnosis: 28

Ran seven half marathons; 2017 Birmingham International Marathon finisher; story featured in Women's Running *magazine; wrote a blog for the Cystic Fibrosis Trust; cystic fibrosis patient and mother to two children, with one having CF*

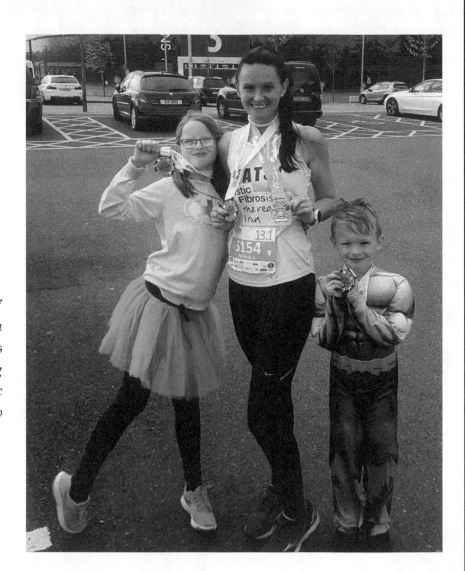

"Those with CF share a deep understanding like no one else ever could."

Natalie Crawford was born prematurely, a very frail, weak baby who failed to thrive. She spent most of her childhood in and out of the hospital with breathing problems, a bad chest, and a constant cough. Doctors diagnosed her with various allergies and asthma, but not cystic fibrosis.

"I missed lots of school and had to fight hard to keep up, struggling to participate in sports due to my body feeling so weak and the constant cough, which wore me out. I decided sports were not for me and instead focused on my studies, unaware of just how crucial staying active was for me."

Natalie's teenage years were filled with recurring bouts of chest infections, which led to pneumonia. But without a diagnosis, let alone a treatment plan and comprehensive lifestyle, her social itinerary included smoky bars, definite red zones for CF patients. "Up until my diagnosis, I believed it was normal to cough up huge amounts of mucus every day and for my sweaty skin to taste so salty," she says.

Then, in 2008, a complicated pregnancy and the premature birth of her first child, Skye-Hope, changed her perspective entirely. "My liver had begun to show signs of decline," says Natalie, "which was then diagnosed as cholestasis, a rare liver condition in pregnancy."

She picked up after her birth and went on to have her second child, Preston, in 2011. "The pregnancy knocked me further into decline, as both my lungs and liver struggled to handle the pressure. At my twenty-week scan, my son was diagnosed with meconium ileus, a blocked bowel. I was told that this was a marker for either cystic fibrosis or Down syndrome, and was offered CVS screening." Tests confirmed her baby boy had cystic fibrosis and that they would need to be transferred to a specialist hospital where they would do Preston's bowel operation soon after birth.

"Genetic counselling was terrifying, and I had never felt so alone in the world. I was offered a termination of my pregnancy, which destroyed me, as I felt that the medical professionals were pushing me into a decision after throwing so many negative facts and statistics at me. The sentence that will always stay in my mind is when they told me my baby would have a poor quality of life, and was that fair, bringing a baby into the world, knowing his life would revolve around hospital admissions?"

Meeting the pediatric CF team who would be caring for her baby was a breath of fresh air for Natalie. "They presented me with the real facts, good and bad, and prepared me for life with CF. We set up a care plan even before Preston was born. I was shown everything that I would have to do to care for him as a newborn, taught physio techniques and medicine regimes.

"Within days, tests confirmed that I, too, had the same mutations as my son. We both had cystic fibrosis." She also learned that her firstborn, Skye, does not have CF, but is a carrier.

"Having a child with CF," she says, "no one will ever understand the fear of passing on to him a deadly bug from one kiss, and the constant worry of the burden we put on our children as we attempt to shield them from the pain we suffer as they help with Mummy's meds, nebulizers, and physio, their tiny hands patting our backs to aid our breathing. This is the hidden part of CF that those without it do not see, our hearts full of fear at the thought of [our children] having to be without us."

Watching her children cope with the disease gave her the strength to endure both her and her son's diagnoses with as much grace as one can muster. "The first year of our [diagnoses] was the hardest," says Natalie, who is also a single parent. But, Preston was born a fighter. "From the moment I held him in my arms, I knew he was strong. And, watching the support and encouragement from his big sister melted me. In Skye, I had another strong little warrior whom I knew would grow to protect her brother, and I was determined to facilitate that bond, which would help us all in the battle we faced."

Natalie says that CF has given her and Preston a bond like no other. "CF is such a lonely condition, as those with CF should not mix due to cross infection. Ironically, the risk that should push [Preston and I] apart forces us closer together, as we share a deep understanding like no one else ever could.

"The sweetest thing is how Preston will always blow his hardest at clinic for his PFTs because he loves to beat my numbers! It is bittersweet that we have to share this journey together—that we make pancakes at 4 a.m. as we snuggle downstairs in our duvet together when our coughing keeps us awake. We take turns patting each other's backs, doing postural drainage. We laugh as we get tangled in each other's nebulizer wires, and share toilet jokes as we both dash to the bathroom when our synchronized 'CF tummy' gives us little warning!"

Natalie says her daughter is also key to their family's success, though she often feels left out because she is the only one of the three not to have the disease. "[Healthy] siblings so often fall under the radar, but our journey is as much hers as it is ours. Skye is the most incredible little nurse for us when we are [sick], and has matured so much faster with extra responsibilities. She is learning to value life and grow up to be thankful, to not judge, and to show empathy to those around her."

Natalie wanted to make an impact on her children's lives while at the same time helping herself. That's what caused her to dive headfirst into researching healthy lifestyles for folks with CF. She came upon the benefits of exercise and the impact it could have on her lungs and her son's—how it could clear the mucus that harbored their nasty infections. "I joined the local gym and started to walk on the treadmill. It was agony. My lungs burnt and I coughed so hard!"

In the background, Natalie had been noticed by

Aaron, one of the personal trainers. "He saw how hard I pushed myself and inquired about my goals. I told him about my diagnosis, and we struck a deal. He was going to teach me how to run, and I was going to beat the life expectancy." Aaron and Natalie agreed on a six-day-a-week training schedule, with Aaron carefully gauging Natalie's progress and gradually increasing her targets.

During this new training regimen, Preston and Natalie both reached first milestones: his first birthday, and her first kilometer on the treadmill. "As I progressed, so did my distances, and I realized that nothing was impossible. With positivity and self-belief, I quickly learned that I could use my running to inspire others, and most importantly, I was determined to make my children proud of me."

Natalie ran her first 5K in 2014 and soon added ten-kilometer races and seven half marathons to her résumé. Then, in October 2017, Natalie did what just a few short years before she would've considered impossible: she ran her first full marathon.

"I love to run, but I love the life that running has given me, and every day I put one foot in front of the other. I am blessed to have my children behind me to be the driving force, the want to succeed."

MERANDA SUE HONAKER

Age: 36

Resides: North Carolina, United States

Age at diagnosis: 18 months

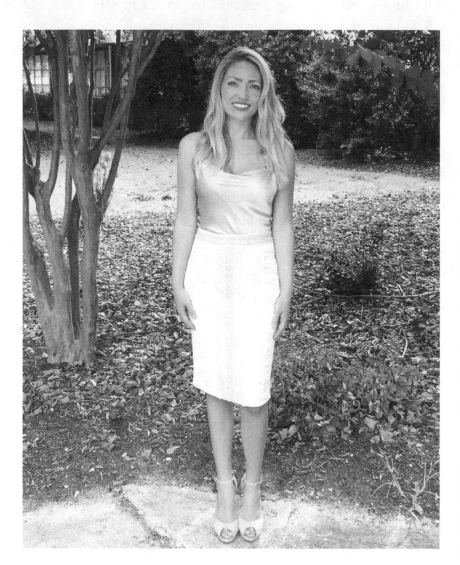

Started her own nonprofit benefiting people with cystic fibrosis called The Salty Life Foundation; served a five-year term with the United States Adult CF Association; founded the Clinical Trials committee; worked with famed CF photographer Ian Pettigrew on The Salty Life: A Cystic Fibrosis Magazine, *where she launched another clinical-trials column within the second publication*

"There is an unsurpassed bond I experience with those affected by CF."

Famed cystic fibrosis warrior and advocate Meranda Sue Honaker grew up in North Carolina in the early eighties, but was not diagnosed with the disease immediately. "I experienced gastrointestinal symptoms, specifically malabsorption, that prompted my mother to seek medical advice." After being told there was nothing wrong with Meranda and to stop bringing her to the local hospital, a nurse pulled her mother aside and encouraged her to take her to the University of North Carolina Hospital for further evaluation. It was there, at eighteen months old, that Meranda was finally diagnosed with cystic fibrosis.

Once diagnosed, Meranda's condition improved. In fact, her first hospitalization was not until she was fifteen years old. "I began to culture a new bacteria, and had been increasingly short of breath. My energy had declined, as well. I spent one month admitted with intravenous antibiotics."

Still, with only one hospitalization in her first fifteen years, Meranda realizes that she was fortunate. "I was exceptionally healthy for a child with CF growing up. CF was not a topic of conversation in my house. My parents were uninformed about CF and the complexities the disease causes. I was told that my pediatric CF doctor told my parents, 'Don't worry about CF. Let her worry about it instead.' I was oblivious to the reality of CF growing up.

"At seventeen, I decided to research cystic fibrosis out of curiosity. I will never forget feeling like my heart had fallen out of my chest when I found out, for the first time, what having CF really meant. I also read the life expectancy at that time, which was utterly heartbreaking for a seventeen-year-old. It was at that moment I decided to devour research, realizing I needed to learn as much as possible to better prepare and understand CF's complications."

Meranda's journey became more difficult when she developed CFRD at seventeen years old after a long course of high-dose steroids resulted in hyperglycemia. After developing CFRD, it became increasingly difficult to manage her health due to more frequent infections. Still, Meranda did not let her health issues stop her from accomplishing her goals. She not only became the first person in her family to graduate high school, but thanks to receiving a full college scholarship awarded by the Boomer Esiason Foundation, she also became the first to graduate college when she earned both her associate's degree in general studies and a bachelor's of science in psychology from the University of Phoenix.

In her early twenties, Meranda developed symptoms of severe nausea, abdominal distention, early satiety (feeling full quickly), and worsening reflux. After three long years, two doctors who misdiagnosed her, and intense suffering on her part, she found a doctor who was able to enroll her in a gastric-emptying study. Shortly after, he diagnosed her with gastroparesis, or delayed gastric emptying. Meranda did her research and outsourced a Canadian promotility drug, which she used for seven years to cure the condition. While she still battles gastric issues like DIOS from time to time, the promotility drug, which she used until 2013, gave her a new lease on life and an understanding that it's up to her to advocate for herself and others with cystic fibrosis.

Meranda spent over fifteen years working with various groups within CF advocating, educating, and serving her community. She has worked tirelessly speaking to and contacting local politicians within North Carolina about the importance of newborn screening and early diagnosis of cystic fibrosis. "Every politician I spoke to was supportive of implementing a newborn-screening law for cystic fibrosis after I explained CF and the positive impact early diagnosis and intervention would bring to those born with the disease."

In January of 2009, thanks to the work of Meranda and many others with the same mission, newborn-screening legislation was passed in North Carolina.

Meranda's biggest contribution to those with cystic fibrosis is her willingness to participate in research. She has participated in over ten clinical trials, most recently completing a two-year safety-and-efficacy study for the newly approved CFTR medication Symdeko, a medication that targets her genetic mutations on a cellular level. "I have been passionate about clinical trials for many years. It is my hope that someday a child born with CF will never endure the struggles of generations past. One way to achieve this is through progress in CF research. I eagerly participate in research studies knowing every study contributes to the greater good of our community. Once a study is complete, data is collected and analyzed, and a decision to pursue FDA approval is made. With every newly approved CF therapy, we are one step closer to our ultimate goal: a cure for all with cystic fibrosis."

In fact, Meranda was recently asked to become an ambassador for the CF Foundation's Clinical Trials Trailblazer campaign, which she calls "a true honor." Her work with clinical trials has earned her the nickname "The CF Trial Warrior."

As proud as she is of her contributions in the CF community, she is most proud of her relationship with her family, specifically her eight-year-old niece, Ava Meranda. Meranda's younger sister, Amanda, named her child after her, a fact that still brings Meranda to tears. "I dress up as Spider-Woman each Halloween and will continue as long as my niece requests it. I love her as my own daughter. I teach her about CF. She knows I have therapies daily, and she enjoys helping me with them. I believe my teaching her about CF will help shape her into a more compassionate person."

Meranda's health over the last year has been a bit more complicated. "After a few years of solid stability, I have spent about twelve weeks on IV antibiotics within the last year. There have been moments of great frustration and struggle. However, I continue persevering, determined to get through it."

Meranda, now thirty-six, was not always confident she would even reach her thirty-fifth birthday. "Now that I [have reached] thirty-five, I am in the bonus rounds of life. Every day I am immensely grateful to continue a beautiful journey in life. Despite CF bringing me immense challenges and sometimes suffering, I never forget how far I have come. I am a resilient, kind-hearted, beautiful woman who loves intensely. My immense love of life and new experiences inspire me every day. Every morning I admire the sunrise as it bathes the earth in such beauty. Life, despite difficulties, is truly beautiful. I want to experience life as profoundly as possible until my last breath."

EMILY SCHALLER

Age: 37

Resides: Michigan, United States

Age at diagnosis: 18 months

Completed fifteen half marathons, several-hundred-mile/cross-state bike rides, a half marathon–distance triathlon, and the 2016 New York City Marathon; started the Rock CF Foundation, which has raised more than $1.5 million and supports research being done by the Cystic Fibrosis Foundation

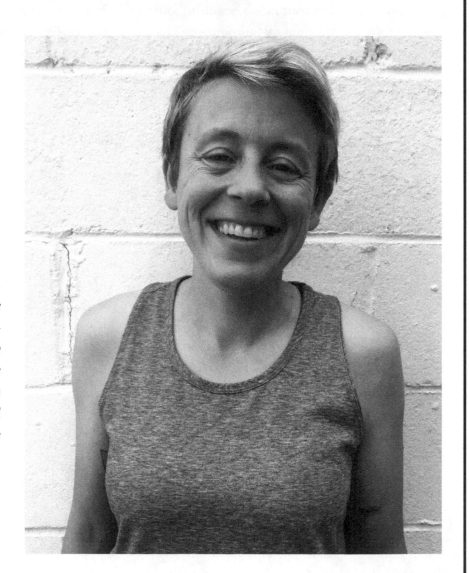

"I was sick of being sick, and knew that there was something that could help me live a better and healthier life."

Some people live to run, but in Emily Schaller's case, she runs to live. The Michigan native had symptoms of failure to thrive and upper respiratory infections during her infancy, but her first sweat test came back negative for CF. However, after her symptoms persisted and Emily had a rectal prolapse, she was tested again at eighteen months. This time the results were positive for cystic fibrosis. Doctors told her parents following the diagnosis that she would probably not survive to the age of eighteen.

Undeterred, her parents were not going to let Emily live in a bubble. "They decided that CF would not dictate any part of our lives." At five, Emily, the youngest of three children and the only one with CF, was displaying her energy by riding around on her skateboard. At nine, she became the starting point guard on her community's basketball team. She attributes the fact that she was active to keeping her out of the hospital until she was thirteen. It was then that the hospitalizations began and she was having lung infections two to three times a year. "My lung function started to decline and I just could not keep up with the other kids as much anymore."

Between the ages of fourteen and seventeen, her health continued to deteriorate. Lung infections were popping up more frequently, and she was being hospitalized two to three times a year. Emily's college career did not last long, as she dropped out of Wayne State University in Detroit after just a

couple of years because she began to believe that her life was going to end soon thanks to CF.

At twenty-two, she was the drummer in an all-girl band that played in smoky bars, further irritating her lungs. Emily says the lowest point was probably in her midtwenties. "I was facing hospitalization after hospitalization and watching my PFTs drop and being okay with it. I was a couch potato, playing drums in smoky bars, and not doing my treatments regularly like I should have been. One day I was out cleaning my car on a nice spring day when suddenly I started to feel my chest tighten and it hurt to take a deep breath. I began feeling weak and I knew something was going on. I was admitted to the hospital with a lung infection, and for the first time in my life I had to wear oxygen for a few days and nights because my O2 [saturation levels] were so low. I didn't know it then, but this was a result of not doing my inhaled meds and vest on a regular basis."

At the age of twenty-five, Emily had had enough. "I was sick of being sick, and knew that there was something that could help me live a better and healthier life."

That "something" was running. Emily began lacing up her shoes, hitting the pavement, and jogging whenever she could. Not only did Emily notice eighteen months free of hospitalizations from her training, but she says that her lung function increased from 50 percent to 70 percent in the three months she began preparing for her first half marathon. She has now completed fifteen half marathons.

A few years later in 2009, Emily was involved in the early trials for Kalydeco. At first she was on the placebo, but eventually doctors put her on the actual drug. She spotted the difference immediately while hanging out with one of her brothers. "We were walking down the street, and I took a deep breath, and when I took a deep breath in and I let it out, I didn't cough. Not only did I not cough, I felt that my lungs were clear and that something huge had happened. It was just something I had never felt in my life before."

Emily soon wanted to become an advocate. "I feel like I have a big voice, and I have to use it to heighten awareness about CF and advocate for clinical trials and a healthy lifestyle." In 2004, she started a rock concert to raise a few dollars and awareness for CF. Three years later, she established a 501(c)(3) organization called the Rock CF Foundation, which is dedicated to increasing the quality of life for people with cystic fibrosis so they can see the same results she has. The foundation utilizes entertainment, fashion, fitness, and the arts to support research initiatives and heighten public awareness in the fight against cystic fibrosis. Her foundation has donated more than five hundred pairs of running shoes to people with cystic fibrosis to inspire them to fight the disease with exercise.

"We created an extensive line of Rock CF merchandise, which is bought by people all over the world because they want to support someone they love with CF. Some of the items do exactly as I dreamed, which is catching the attention of groups of people who have no connection to CF, like runners and fitness gurus. They love the design, buy it, and then learn about Rock CF and what CF is. With this, we are opening a door into the CF world."

The Rock CF Foundation has also raised more than $1.5 million and supports research being done by the Cystic Fibrosis Foundation. Rock CF's funding also supports its own Kicks Back program, EmPower program with Attain Health, grants for advocacy, sponsorships for other CF nonprofits, and its own line of merchandise, which is its largest awareness platform. The foundation even has its own annual race south of Detroit called the Rock CF Rivers Half Marathon, which brings 2,500 runners together to support Emily's charity. Emily calls the participants part of her "Rock CF army."

Emily continues to practice what she preaches by raising awareness along with her "exercise hero" and CF cohort, Jerry Cahill. The two of them biked both cross-country and internationally to raise funds and awareness for the Boomer Esiason Foundation, while also demonstrating the importance of exercise for someone with CF as part of Bike to Breathe since 2014. And, in 2016, Emily ran the New York City Marathon, a feat she never imagined she could accomplish. "That is something I will never forget. The energy was sky high, and I felt like I was running in the clouds the whole time."

Today this thirty-seven-year-old Michigander continues to raise awareness through her foundation. Emily runs about twenty-five miles a week during her nonmarathon training and currently thirty to forty miles a week as she trains to run her third marathon in Chicago in October 2019.

"I've never been happier or healthier and look at each mile as my fight against CF!"

KATIE MALIK

Age: 37

Resides: Washington State, United States

Age at diagnosis: 2

Professional opera singer; starred on the international Emmy Award™–winning TV reality series **Allt för Sverige** *(Great Swedish Adventure); received a grant from the Cystic Fibrosis Foundation to spearhead a new program called CF Yogi, which is creating a virtual yoga studio for the CF community*

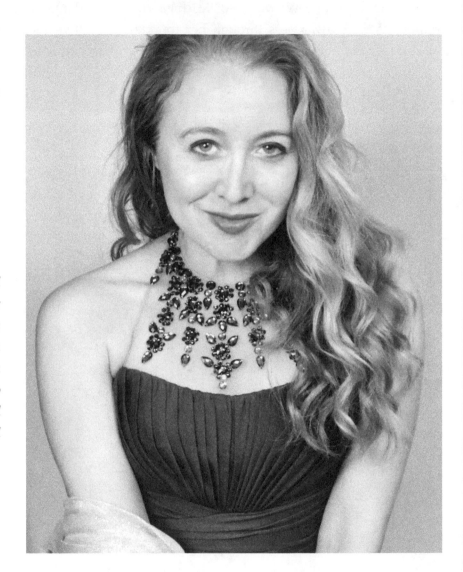

"It's not about being 'fearless,' it's about pushing past the wall of fear because of all the possibilities that are waiting for you on the other side."

CF has presented opera singer Katie Malik with many challenges as an artist. Symptoms like sinusitis, mucus congestion, and an incessant cough, which sometimes requires IV cleanouts, add a daunting dimension to the Olympic feat—the discipline, focus, stamina, and years of training—of singing in a three-hour opera. But, Katie has learned how to manage, and she's discovered that in spite of those challenges, performing in opera is actually one of the things she does best.

The doctors knew there was something wrong with Katie from the time that she was six months old—she was simply failing to thrive—but it took a long time to get the correct diagnosis. Her parents were very supportive of her growing up and encouraged her to do the things she loved, which included not only singing, but dancing and competing in archery tournaments with her dad.

"My attitude toward CF as a kid wasn't a particularly involved one. I was always pretty healthy, and so it wasn't a huge deal to me. I did know that there were shortened life expectancies, and I thought about my own mortality more than most kids probably do, but I didn't think of myself as 'sick,' and lived an otherwise pretty normal childhood. I had to go to the doctor a lot, but I didn't have any big defining moments around CF when I was a kid." Katie credits singing for keeping her so healthy.

Katie's first real scare with CF occurred when she was twenty years old and a junior at Seattle Pacific University, where she received both academic and music scholarships. "I had my first episode of hemoptysis shortly after the fall quarter started," says Katie. "It was terrifying to me. I was just getting ready to go out with friends to a campus event, felt that I had to cough, and went to the bathroom. Seeing pure, bright-red blood in the sink felt like an out-of-body experience. I'd never been hospitalized before and I was feeling fine, so it really came as a shock.

"I had to stay a couple of days in the hospital and then did home IV antibiotics in my campus apartment for a couple of weeks. During Christmas break, the same thing happened again without warning, and I was scared that this was somehow going to be the 'new normal.' Luckily, I haven't been hospitalized since then, though I have had other episodes of hemoptysis and been on home IVs about once per year."

Katie graduated from Seattle Pacific magna cum laude in the University Scholars honors program. Since college, Katie's become an opera singer and yoga instructor. "I've performed with a professional opera company, Tacoma Opera, since 2008," she says. "I became a regular chorister, and in 2013 I made my solo debut as Edith in the *Pirates of Penzance*. Subsequent roles have included the Cousin in Puccini's *Madame Butterfly* and Betty in Kurt Weill's *The Threepenny Opera*. I've also begun working as a choreographer for the company, for the aforementioned *Threepenny Opera*, and the upcoming production of Franz Lehar's *The Merry Widow*."

Katie performs in two opera productions in the US per year, on average, and has also performed in international venues as far away as Thailand. She recently began performing with the CF Virtual Choir, a group of CF singers who perform together virtually in order to avoid bacterial cross-contamination. Their first project was featured on an album called "Stand Together" by Choirs with Purpose, which was endorsed by Sir Paul McCartney and became a contender for the number-one Christmas album in the UK.

Katie says that having CF can be a tug-of-war between the simultaneous desires to be treated as if she does not have CF, yet still be acknowledged for what she has accomplished despite of it. "I want my singing to be considered alongside others without CF so that my work stands on its own merits," she says. "In fact, for many years I kept my CF quiet so that casting directors would not know about it, but would consider me on the same-level playing field as everyone else. I don't want to be given a 'handicap' or extra consideration.

"Yet, I also need a certain level of accommodation and grace given. Sometimes my schedule requires me to take a break for my nebs before I sing, or I have to eat when other people don't. So, while on one hand I don't want people to know about it and make a big fuss, on the other I also want them to know about it and give me the benefit of the doubt that I'm not asking for anything I don't genuinely need."

In 2014, Katie was on the international Emmy-winning TV reality series *Allt för Sverige* (Great Swedish Adventure), which she describes as *The Amazing Race* meets *Who Do You Think You Are?* They take Americans with Swedish heritage around Sweden to learn about their roots and ancestry. There are competitions in each episode, and the loser has to leave. The grand prize is a reunion with your long-lost Swedish relatives.

Katie believes that CF might have gotten her on the show. "Since CF is a genetic disease, and I don't have any family members with the disease, I was curious to find out where my CF came from and whether I had any living relatives with CF in Sweden. I mentioned that in my audition video, and the producers were very curious to hear about CF and its role in my life as a singer and how the shortened life expectancy impacted my life and the decisions I've made. When they cast me on the show, we had to take into account the filming and travel schedule and how I would fit my treatments into the production of the show. While there was a lot that we had to manage behind the scenes, it didn't end up impacting my performance in any of the competitions, and the audience wound up rooting for me, as I became something of a fan-favorite underdog.

"As a singer I was always a little leery of talking about my CF publicly, but once I committed to doing the show and owning my story, there was such an outpouring of love and support that I was happy that I made the decision to open up about it."

As runner-up, Katie made it all the way to the final challenge. Though she missed out on the grand prize, she was invited back for an all star–style Christmas special where she did get to meet her relatives and celebrate Christmas with them. Today, Katie and her relatives have become very good friends. Her season (season 4 in 2014) had the highest ratings in the show's history, and the finale was watched by two million people in a country of nine million.

"I subsequently returned to Sweden and completed a solo concert tour in many of Sweden's beautiful churches, including the historic Lund Cathedral. While I was in the country, I also completed an independent summit of Sweden's highest mountain, Kebnekaise.'"

About eight years ago, Katie developed a new passion upon discovering yoga during a period of illness where her lung function unexpectedly dropped about 20 percent. "It had always been in the high sixty to seventy percent range, and dropped to almost fifty percent during one exacerbation. I committed myself to exercising at least thirty minutes a day, every day, no excuses, and decided to try every exercise class at my local gym to find out what I liked and what I would stick with. I also decided to make myself a guinea pig and measured my FEV1 on my home spirometer, and charted the results in Excel. I noticed a trend—on days when I did yoga, singing, or hiking, I had higher FEV1 that night and the next morning. So, I started focusing more on those things.

"Through a combination of IV antibiotics and exercise, I regained that lost lung function within six months. Yoga is powerful because it taught me to recognize that letting go of expectations is a powerful and beautiful thing. When you let go of your preconceptions, you're also letting go of the limits you've placed on yourself. You find out that your world is bigger than you thought it was."

Katie soon began teaching at community gyms. Soon, she developed a series of "Yoga for CF" videos for the Cystic Fibrosis Trust in collaboration with an online fitness platform called Pactster, which hosts customized workouts for unique medical conditions. In the fall of 2018, the Cystic Fibrosis Foundation announced Katie as one of the new Impact Grant recipients. She is now spearheading a new program called CF Yogi, which is creating a virtual yoga studio for the CF community.

"You have to have something you want to do in order to make a change. Find the passion that drives you, and set a goal that's just out of your reach. Identify the obstacles in your way and work past or around them. I've found that the changes I've feared the most are the ones that I most needed to make. It's not about being 'fearless,' it's about pushing past the wall of fear because of all the possibilities that are waiting for you on the other side."

JAMES CAMERON

Age: 39

Resides: Burlington, Ontario, Canada

Age at diagnosis: 5 months

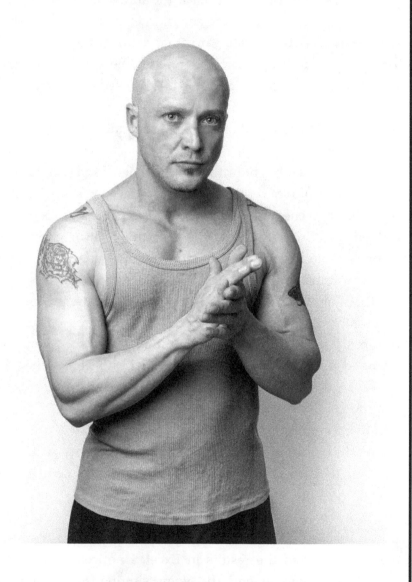

Won two gold medals in long jump and shot-put, and a bronze medal in triples lawn bowling at the Canadian Transplant Games in the summer of 2016 at the age of thirty-six; competes on a dragon boat team consisting of transplant recipients and living donors that, over the past five years, has won multiple gold, silver, and bronze medals; competed in combat sports

"Having a double-lung transplant is the closest thing to heaven without actually dying."

The Terminator is a 1984 film directed by James Cameron about a seemingly indestructible force played by Hollywood and bodybuilding icon Arnold Schwarzenegger. Our story, though, is about a different James Cameron. This legendary CF warrior also happens to be a virtually unbeatable force whose hero just happens to be Arnold Schwarzenegger. James, in fact, met his hero in 2013, months before beginning his own journey in bodybuilding.

James is 5'7" and weighs in around 152 pounds. This chiselled gladiator survived seven near-fatal infections, four life-saving operations, and dramatically improved his quality of life by implementing two key elements into his lifestyle: fitness and nutrition. "I want to inspire people to do the same, so they experience the satisfaction it brings."

James remembers his school days quite vividly. "Gym class was tough, trying to keep up with my peers, at first," he says. "I wanted so badly to be equal among them, if not better, so I started to get in shape at home doing sit-ups while doing my mask/nebulizer treatment, doing wall push-ups until I could do bed push-ups, then finally regular push-ups off the floor. Same with chin-ups. These simple workouts on a daily basis helped me be good at whatever challenge was thrown at me."

James was not the biggest kid growing up and was bullied a few times. He leaned on his uncle, a boxer who grew up in Poland. He understood the fight ahead for James and decided to give him tools that would serve him throughout his life against anyone who might pick on him. He taught James at the age of ten how to box and defend himself.

"If, by chance, I were cornered, there's either fight or flight. I chose to fight. It made me a stronger person." Eventually, James became an amateur boxer himself, while also competing in karate and judo. He accumulated about a hundred wins in just four years.

While his uncle played a key role in his life, James says it was his parents who established the foundation of an open mind, allowing him to do something as seemingly dangerous as boxing in the first place. "My parents let me experience everything that piqued my interest," he says. They also made eating healthy paramount in his upbringing. "Nutrition has never been a problem for me," says James. "My mother is an exceptional cook. Growing up, she ruled the kitchen with an iron fist. She was on par for everything CF related, and even fought the doctors on high-calorie diet choices. Every meal was healthy before and after my ascension into fitness. The only thing I've ever had to worry about was taking my CF enzymes."

James, born in Canada, has dual citizenship both there and in Poland. He says his first brush with the scariness of CF came when he was just shy of his thirteenth birthday on a return trip from visiting family in Poland in 1992. He had his first hospital admittance upon returning from the trip. The hospitalization lasted about six weeks. "I went to my CF clinic, and they told me my PFTs were down and my sputum looked horrible," he says. "It was the first time I was told those dreaded words all CF warriors fear: 'You won't be going home today!' It was the first time I was taken away from my comfortable everyday life. From that point on, I call [hospital stays] 'CF prison,' because you leave your pets, family, home, friends, everything. They come to visit during visiting hours. Your meals come on time, as do the medication and physio sessions."

James eventually left the hospital and did his best to stay in shape. At age fourteen, he added bodybuilding-style weight training to his regular gym routine, which featured push-ups, squats, and lots of skipping. As James got older, though, his lung function began to deteriorate—so much so that doctors told him he had to have a double-lung transplant, otherwise he'd have about two weeks to live.

"At the end of my end-stage CF, me, being as stubborn as can be, kept refusing to sign papers for double-lung transplantation. I thought I could beat this infection—beat this end-stage CF that the docs kept talking about. As more time went by, my window of opportunity began to dwindle, and my pride just wouldn't let go. My team of doctors said that if I didn't get this transplant, my feeble fourteen percent lung capacity wasn't going to last much longer. Still, I refused to agree to the procedure."

James' family surprised him with an intervention. "I'm in a room full of people," he says, "and my mother hands me some papers to sign. I put my initials down so those papers can be processed. After everybody had gone home, I cried. I felt like I threw in the towel and had given up my fight. I had a specific routine I created to heal myself in times like this that had worked so many times, but this time it was like trying to push a boulder up a mountain. But, after a few hours, I felt at peace, like a feeling of knowing everything will be okay. No more fear, no more nervousness. I just let go and put my trust into other people's hands. My lung capacity dropped down to eleven percent in less than a few days. Now, this is what shocked my world—only five days after signing to be on the transplant waiting list, I got my call for lungs!"

At twenty-four years old, he underwent the strenuous but lifesaving procedure. "Having a double-lung transplant is the closest thing to heaven without actually dying," he says, meaning getting new lungs is like being able to breathe freely, how regular people do. "My only regret about end-stage CF is not signing my name on those transplant papers sooner. So much time wasted in agony, when I could have felt healthy much sooner."

Following his transplant, James began his comeback. With a lung capacity almost double his pretransplant baseline, James could pretty much do anything he wanted. He remembers going to the beach shortly after his stint in the hospital and running so fast that, for once, his legs tired before his lungs. He hired a coach and got back into bodybuilding training. His girlfriend, Jackie, whom he calls "Nurse Jackie" because of how much she has taken care of him over the years, motivated him to do it. Training consisted of boxing cardio in the morning and weightlifting every evening.

"I competed in bodybuilding as a bucket-list write-off in 2013," he says. "That turned into qualifying to compete at the Canadian Provincials bodybuilding show in 2014. After Provincials, I qualified for the Canadian Nationals in body-building in Quebec in the fall of 2014." James also earned a place in the *Guinness Book of World Records* when, as part of a team representing Canada in a caber-tossing event, eighty simultaneous throwers flipped sixty-nine cabers, making Canada the world-record holder.

James is passionate about CF awareness, and used his profile to write an article for the first edition of *Cystic Fibrosis* magazine in 2016. He also took part in a commercial campaign for organ donation, #theorganproject, which was filmed at Toronto General Hospital in the summer of 2016.

During his impressive run of athletic accomplishments, James came up with TrainLikeMe, a program that prepares someone with CF for the worst to come. "I share routines and nutrition plans I created based on the ultrasensitivity that we have when we are in the hospital. I've always been the kind of guy that puts hard work into the gym," he says, "and I love to show or teach by example. If you want to learn something, you can either read it in a book, watch it on YouTube, or put some gym clothes on and grind it out with me!"

And he doesn't reserve this attitude for the weight room. "In public places, I let people see me self-inject with insulin and take handfuls of pills before a large meal," he says. "I've never been in a position where I felt uncomfortable. I think of it as, this person might never run into another one of us again, so be kind and leave a good first impression."

While he spends much of his time connecting with the global CF community, he continues to mentor five-hundred-plus people living with the disease, offering tips, advice, and promoting healthy living for a much stronger cystic fibrosis family.

James says his fight against CF has not been a fight he's been in alone. Besides his amazing family, he praises Jackie. "By definition, she's a soul mate—the kind of person who knows what you're thinking before having to say it—the kind of person who knows something is wrong, and how to make it better. She is nothing short of phenomenal."

James says that CF will mentally challenge you every single day. "If you can live through a week with CF, you can consider yourself a mental magician. If you miss a dose, miss a treatment, miss a meal, you will pay for it. But, if you put in the work, keep up with everything, you will be on top of the world."

Just ask CF's version of *The Terminator*!

KC WHITE

Age: 40

Resides: Ohio, United States

Age at diagnosis: 3

Recipient of both the Cystic Fibrosis Foundation Alex Award and Boomer Esiason Foundation Michael Brennan Courage Award; co-chair of the first BreatheCon; chair of the Cystic Fibrosis Foundation's Adult Advisory Council; serves on the National Board of Trustees for the Cystic Fibrosis Foundation

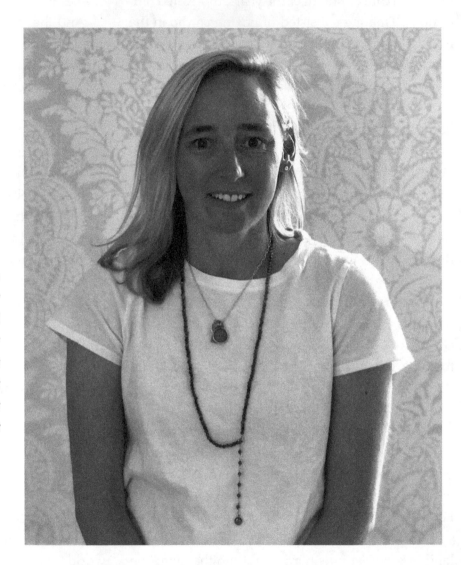

"I very much believe playing sports helped me stay healthy more than anything else."

When KC White was twenty-two, she went to every major-league baseball stadium and threw out the first pitches to raise awareness and funds for CF. Her first-pitch awareness campaign became known as the Tour for a Cure and was documented in *USA Today* and several other newspapers across the country. She was even invited on to *Good Morning America*. KC has been doing "pitches" most of her life to raise money for CF, but her journey did not begin until the age of three.

When KC was born in Charlotte, North Carolina, her doctors thought her common cold symptoms were just allergies. KC believes the doctors decided not to do further testing because antibiotics like Bactrim® always seemed to mitigate the symptoms. Her parents suspected there was more to the story.

Her family moved to Buffalo, New York, when she was three for her dad's job. There, at Women's and Children's Hospital, pulmonologist Dr. Michelle Cloutier knew within five minutes to diagnose KC with CF.

Before she was diagnosed, like so many CF babies, KC was failing to thrive. However, once she started taking enzymes at the age of three, she was much more active and vibrant. "Raise KC to be a responsible adult," Dr. Cloutier advised her parents. She believed KC would outlive childhood. This was a brave assertion for the early 1980s, but she was encouraged by both KC's response to the enzymes and advances in research, which would eventually lead to the pivotal discovery of the cystic fibrosis gene in 1989.

Dr. Cloutier had one other request: "Get [KC] involved in sports." So, KC joined a swim team at age four and a soccer team at age five. While her mom even petitioned the school for extra gym classes to keep KC in shape, administrators appeared to make an exception just for her. "I remember playing games and running in the gym with my gym teacher while the rest of my classmates were reading in the classroom," KC recalls. "I thought having CF was kind of awesome in that moment."

She went on to earn ten varsity letters in high school in soccer, basketball, and crew. Then, in college, she played club soccer, basketball, roller hockey, and softball. "I very much believe playing sports helped me stay healthy more than anything else," says KC. "I didn't have to do airway clearance until adulthood because of sports."

When her own amateur athletic career was over, she served as head varsity lacrosse coach at Chagrin Falls High School in Chagrin Falls, Ohio, a small town outside Cleveland, for eight years. Before retiring in 2017, KC led her team to the final four seven times, the state finals four times, and was named US Lacrosse North Coast Chapter Coach of the Year in 2016.

KC's incredible drive and personality were recognized early. At only four years old, she became involved with the CF Foundation through a letter campaign her grandmother started called the KC Bryan Life Fund. The fund managed to raise thousands of dollars each year in honor of her granddaughter. KC's grandparents also started the CF Sports Challenge in Cleveland, which ran for twenty years, some years raising more than $100,000 annually for the CF Foundation. KC handed out medals to the winning teams each year, and eventually gave her first speech there when she was just nine. Between the KC Bryan Life Fund and the CF Sports Challenge, KC's grandparents have raised millions for the Cystic Fibrosis Foundation.

Since her first speech, KC has been regularly called upon to advocate. She has had the honor of speaking at many CFF and BEF (Boomer Esiason Foundation) events over her lifetime, and is a recognizable face at CFF's signature Great Strides walk.

The community of people with whom she has connected have backed her tremendously, as evidenced by the $250,000 raised by her Friends of KC National Family Team.

KC lives in Chagrin Falls with Justin, her husband of fifteen years, and their twelve-year-old son, Mac.

"I had a long time to think about [KC], the disease, and all that comes with it," says Justin. "As our relationship grew, it became clear that she was the person I wanted to spend my life with. CF played almost no role in my decision by that time. I honestly think dating and marrying someone with a terminal illness requires the right kind of person. If you are a person that gets stressed out by life's every little detail, you might need to reconsider. It doesn't mean you are a bad person or a weak person. It just means you are probably going to struggle mightily in the relationship and it might not be a good idea. I appreciate every second with KC and Mac. As much as she uses me for support, I use her to learn to appreciate life more, to not sweat the small stuff. I think we are even."

Justin and KC not only live for each other, but also for Mac. KC does not plan on going anywhere despite the tough times that CF often brings.

"I intend to witness all [Mac's] milestones—his graduations, his wedding, his children."

CHRIS DAVIES

Age: 40   **Resides:** Adelaide, South Australia, Australia   **Age at diagnosis:** 6 months

Chris is a retired professional Premier Cricket player. He is also the second-ever recipient of the Tanya Denver award, given to an Australian sportsman or sportswoman for outstanding sportsmanship and endeavor. Chris, former general manager of operations of the Australian Cricketers' Association and former general manager of football at the South Australian National Football League, is the current general manager of football operations at the Port Adelaide Football Club in the Australian Football League (AFL).

"Life is not measured by the number of breaths we take, but by the moments that take our breath away."

SOMER LOVE

Age: 40

Resides: Utah, United States

Age at diagnosis: 11 months

Spreads her positive message through social media and her blog; created Love To Breathe® in 2001; she and her family were instrumental in starting the Utah chapter of the CF Foundation while starting Taste of Utah, which has raised over $3.5 million for the CF Foundation; participates with a parent-advisory council and meets with CF parents regularly to discuss life and strategies to stay healthy; 2019 recipient of the Cystic Fibrosis Foundation Alex Award

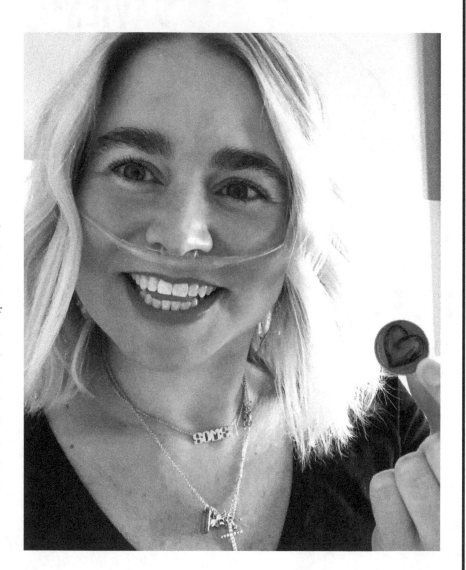

"CF is a blessing in an ugly disguise."

The aptly named Somer Love can take even the scariest things and make them seem comical. Take her lung x-rays, for instance, which she calls her "pearly whites." Over time, her lung function has deteriorated to below 30 percent. "My lungs are on a slow but steady decline," she sighs with resolve. "I try not to focus on the numbers too much. While that's easier said than done, the mind can be a powerful healing tool, and I will continue to breathe through my battlefield and do everything in my power to survive, because surviving is my reality."

Somer's parents set the tone for her inspiring attitude. "I was diagnosed one month before I turned one," she says, "so my parents threw me a huge birthday party. Every birthday is so important to me. That first birthday definitely set the tone for how we try to celebrate each year."

Appropriately, she shares her spirit with children by being a mentor to her younger peers. "I love being there for the younger generation," she says. "CF is so isolating, and the only way to truly escape that isolation, I think, is by surrounding yourself with people that just 'get it.' I hope seeing an older peer going through the same challenging treatments and maintaining a positive attitude will help them to do the same."

Somer has expanded her passion through a mission she calls Love To Breathe, which she created in 2001 to spread positive energy to the CF community, specifically families with newly diagnosed children. "I want to spread love and CF awareness, and give hope to everyone I encounter."

Somer spreads her positive message through her blog, social media, and her personal favorite, her Love To Breathe Tokens. "I created the Love To Breathe Token in 2014 in hopes of changing the world, or at least doing my part to make a positive impact." While the tokens do not have any monetary value, Somer hopes their worth will mean much more than that. "My goal was to create something that could spread more love in a world that so desperately needs it, and at the same time spread awareness for cystic fibrosis. The front of the token is my logo that I painted, and on the back, it says, 'Keep It, Pass It, Hold It Close, whatever you choose to do, love will follow it through.'"

The tokens are now circulating in over seventy countries and all fifty states. That's about 30 percent of the world!

"Knowing that each token has had an impact on someone means the world to me. I love checking the hashtag #LoveToBreatheTokens and seeing the fun pics that people have taken all over the world to spread love and CF awareness."

Somer is unequivocal about the fact that "CF has made me stronger, fight harder, love more, and truly appreciate life, one breath at a time. CF is a blessing in an ugly disguise. It's my reality, and it has made me who I am today. For that, I really am grateful."

INKA NISINBAUM

Age: 40

Resides: Missouri, United States

Age at diagnosis: Birth

Motivational speaker; author of two books with a third on the way; the first woman worldwide to have a baby after a double-lung-and-liver transplant

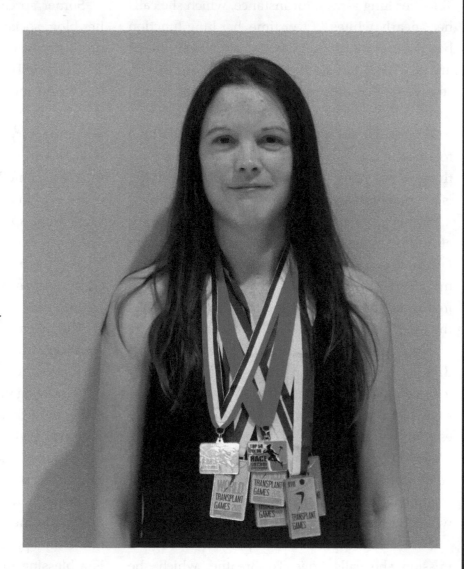

"I don't want to worry what will be in two, five, or ten years. I'm here today, and that's all that matters."

Inka Nisinbaum was born on March 17, 1979, in Germany with meconium ileus. A five-hour operation on her second day of life saved her, but her diagnosis was clear: cystic fibrosis. Her doctors predicted a life expectancy of four years.

"Obviously, my doctors were wrong," says Inka. "I grew up almost unaffected by my disease until I reached the age of ten, when CF slowly started to catch up to me. My lung function was around seventy-five percent before I had more and more lung infections and was diagnosed with the beginnings of liver cirrhosis. I had my first month-long hospital stay and my first IV antibiotic therapy."

During this time, Inka's dad got her into running. He wanted to help her loosen the phlegm in her lungs because Inka, who was ten at the time, was coughing a lot more than normal.

"I [joined] a running club, and I was a pretty good runner. I won trophies and was proud being a successful member of a team, especially since I was running with and against healthy teens. It became my therapy and literally saved my life," says Inka, who was running three miles a day four to five times a week with her dad by the age of ten.

"Running enabled me to get all the mucus out of my lungs. It strengthened my breathing muscles, improved my overall fitness and my resilience. It kept me breathing for much longer than expected."

As Inka made the transition to living on her own and going to college, she did less competing, instead running just to stay healthy. Soon, though, running became close to impossible for Inka because she developed ascites, an abnormal buildup of water in the abdomen, caused by her failing liver. "Running became a struggle. I remember one run specifically. I was running at a park when suddenly a man in a suit and a suitcase bypassed me. He wasn't running. He was just walking fast. This was the moment when I realized that running was not an option anymore. I stopped running soon after, a decision that caused my lungs to decline, as well.

"My doctors saw the decline in my health way before me. At least a year passed before I realized that I needed a transplant. My doctors were already talking about it, making me shake my head because I thought, 'A transplant? That's for really sick people, not for me.'"

Things unfortunately got even worse for Inka. "At the age of twenty-two, I was told I had one last chance—a double-lung-and-liver transplant. I waited fifteen months for my transplant, in which I came a couple of times close to death."

Inka remembers getting the phone call informing her that her team had found a donor. "I was excited and relieved. I didn't want the life I had at that time—this life of not being able to breathe, of sitting at home, living again with my parents. I wanted a second chance or no life at all, and that phone call granted me that second chance."

Inka was transplanted on December 28, 2002.

When she woke up from her surgery, she felt horrible. "I stayed intubated (still had a breathing tube) for four days after my transplant. When they finally allowed me to breathe on my own, and allowed me to wake up, I wasn't able to breathe because I had lost my breathing muscles, and all my other muscles, as well. I was not able to lift my head on my own at that time. I was that weak."

Due to her difficulty breathing and all the meds that were in her system, Inka thought she only got a new liver and still had her old lungs. Only when the doctor, who got the organs for her, came to visit her a day later did she understand that she had survived a double-lung-and-liver transplant.

"After my organ transplant, I struggled to connect with life again. During this time, I always said God had sent me back, but forgot to tell me why."

Then Inka found an old ritual that changed her mindset. "I knew that running could help me. Now, running helps me to believe in my health. When I doubt it, I run, because when I run, I feel strong, I feel resilient, and most of all, I feel healthy. That's why I run."

Soon after finding her love for running again, the rest of Inka's life began to take shape. She was having coffee with friends, shopping without coughing or running out of breath, going back to her university, and being able to live by herself again. "By cherishing the healthy components of my life, and not dwelling on the disabled ones, I fought my way back to life."

In November of 2005, a few years after her transplant, Inka was at a dance club in Germany when a gentleman named Nadav asked for her number. After two years together, the couple were married in September of 2007.

Despite having a triple organ transplant, she and Nadav wanted to have a baby. "We were warned about having a baby," says Inka. "The risks of me getting pregnant were just countless. And nobody knew how it would work out after a double-lung-and-liver transplant, because no one ever had a baby after this kind of transplant. And of course, we were scared, as well, especially me. I knew how hard I had to fight to get where I was. Was I ready to risk all of that for a baby? I think for my husband, it was a little bit easier to decide. He had never seen me sick. We met after my transplant. To him, I was a triple-organ-transplant recipient, but healthy. My husband was confident, more or less, right from the start. I needed more time to say yes and feel confident with my answer."

Inka and Nadav started their "journey called pregnancy" in Germany in 2006, where none of Inka's doctors wanted to support their decision. "Same in Austria, where we lived for two years," says Inka, "and also here in the US, the only feedback we got when we started to talk about pregnancy was 'no' and 'you could die.' I was ready to give up when one doctor in St. Louis showed slight support. He was at least ready to discuss a potential pregnancy, and that gave me all the hope and support I needed to eventually say yes. We moved to Dallas, and we somehow found the right team of doctors that gave us the confidence we needed to give it a try."

Through IVF, Inka became pregnant in 2013. "My pregnancy was surprisingly normal," she says. "I only had two complications. The first, in the beginning of the pregnancy, was when I almost got a bowel obstruction. It was taken care of via enemas and me walking in the gym on the treadmill. The second was toward the end, around the thirty-second week. The fetus was growing and therefore pushing up my bowel, but my bowel was stuck and wouldn't move up due to inner scar tissue. I spent one night in the delivery room, got two morphine drips that allowed me to sleep, and in the morning, my husband and I drove back home. I was still in excruciating pain, but day after day the scar tissue loosened, and eventually the pain was gone. My son was born in 2013 full term via C-section. Tiny, but completely healthy."

Today, Inka can say she is a healthy CF patient and triple-organ-transplant recipient, and she is the first woman worldwide who has had a baby after a double-lung-and-liver transplant. "My donor didn't just save me, but the next generation, too," she says. Today, her son, Noam, is five years old, which is significant since her family was told Inka would not live to that same age.

Inka is healthier than she has been in a long time. The few times she has been to the doctor, Nadav has been by her side. "He's fighting with doctors, brings coffee to the hospital, sits with all the moms at playgrounds so our son can play no matter what, and makes stupid jokes once I'm able to laugh again."

Inka knows that without her husband she would not have the life that she has now. "Nadav is the biggest believer in my health and my abilities. He always believed I would be able to have a child, do anything I want, but when I'm down he also understands the severity of it, and knows how to handle it."

Inka now wants to spread confidence to others the way her husband has done for her. She is now a motivational speaker who speaks frequently in both Germany and the United States. The couple lives in St. Louis, Missouri.

"I'm healthy now," Inka says, as she has now resumed her three-mile runs while still caring for Noam. "I do what I can and believe in staying healthy, and just take it one day after another. I don't want to worry what will be in two, five, or ten years. I don't want to live with a death sentence over my head that calls itself a prognosis. I'm here today, and that's all that matters."

TIM SWEENEY

Age: 42

Resides: Connecticut, United States

Age at diagnosis: 2

Husband; father of three children: Timmy, Harrison, and Finn; double-lung-transplant recipient; personal trainer; 2010 finisher of the New York City Marathon

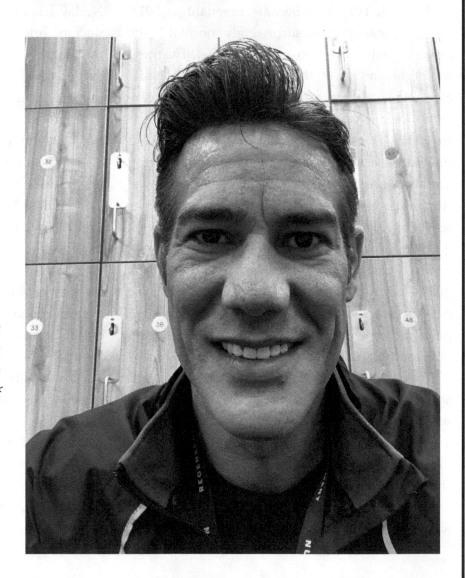

"Here I was, running in the biggest marathon in the world next to the man who had saved me."

Some consider Superman a guy who dons a cape and leaps over tall buildings. Those people have not met Tim Sweeney, whose Instagram handle and website are, in fact, titled *The Everyday Superman* because of the way he fights cystic fibrosis.

On November 10, 2009, Tim was still trying to breathe on his own. He remembers waking up in the ICU just hours after an emergency double-lung transplant. There, he noticed his surgeon, Dr. Joshua Sonett, limping around the room.

"I asked him why he was limping. He said that it was from the New York City Marathon he had just run. I told him that was something I would love to do someday, and he said that we should do it together next year. I took him up on his offer."

Tim had never been a long-distance runner, and running a marathon, much less one of the biggest marathons in the world, was not on his bucket list. "But when Dr. Sonett said that I could do it, something just clicked." Tim didn't take Dr. Sonett's comment as a joke; he took it to mean that he thought Tim would be able and ready to run almost thirty miles in less than twelve months. Tim was motivated to leave the hospital and start training.

Tim's journey prior to his transplant began nearly three decades earlier. At two years of age, he was diagnosed with cystic fibrosis. Yet, Tim never knew he had cystic fibrosis, despite his early diagnosis. His parents, Russell and Rosemarie, kept it from him to keep him normal. Rosemarie told him later on, "We didn't want to give you a label."

To this day, Tim does not blame his parents. "I would have handled it the same way."

He never missed any school and did all of the proper treatments. He never thought of himself as terminally ill, just that he always had a "cold" and had to take enzymes to make him better. "I always knew there was something different when I grew up. I always had a slight cough in the morning, but as the day went on, it became less and less," Tim said.

His parents got Tim into exercise to battle the disease. It was actually Rosemarie who encouraged him, and Russell who got him started. "My dad was an athlete. He often took me on training runs on the road or by bike. It got me excited about exercise.

"My father bought me a weight set for the basement, as well as a heavy bag and whatever else gym equipment I asked for. We ran in road races together, but by twelve I could not run anymore. This is when I switched over to anaerobic sports like racquetball and tennis."

In high school, Tim lost the passion for endurance sports because he didn't like the way it made his lungs feel. So, he focused more on lifting weights. At twenty-one, Tim entered his first bodybuilding show. He came in fifth in the men's division and second in the junior division. The guy who won the men's division turned out to be future WWE star John Cena.

That same year, Tim lost his father, his role model. "I believe our parents teach us through their actions and behaviors. When my father was hired by the fire department, I was a few months old. He was in a bad motorcycle accident and lost his right patella. Doctors said he would never walk right again. He proved them wrong when he rehabbed himself through exercise and walking. He would walk around town with a cane and tears in his eyes through the pain. He not only walked again, but he became a great athlete afterward, and a firefighter. This was the role model I had. Never give up."

Tim graduated college and became a personal trainer. It wasn't until his wife, Beth, heard something in his chest in 2004, when he was in his midtwenties, that he got the official diagnosis from the doctor. "They asked, 'How long have you known you had cystic fibrosis?' and I was like, 'Whoa!' It was a major shock." Still, Tim was actually relieved to know what he was up against.

In 2007, his health began to decline. Tim and Beth were able to have a baby boy, Timmy, through in-vitro fertilization, but doctors told Tim if he did not get a lung transplant, his days would end in the next eighteen months. That's when he was introduced to Dr. Sonett.

In the fall of 2009, Tim could not even walk across a room without an oxygen mask due to his CF. Fighting double pneumonia while losing his hair, a ton of weight, and 80 percent of his lung function, Tim needed help fast. Another infection would probably kill him. Still, Tim wasn't giving up. That's when Dr. Sonett began making his presence felt in Tim's life. He told Tim, "If you're walking into the transplant, you're walking out after." So, Tim lifted light weights in his hospital room and walked as much as he could down the hospital corridor.

In preparation of his surgery, his family chipped in and bought a treadmill for his basement. Everyone was setting Tim up for success. All that was left was getting him his new lungs and a second chance at life. When the donor finally became available, Dr. Sonett performed the transplant.

Now, it was time to train for the New York City Marathon and live up to his end of the deal. The second day after his surgery, Tim walked to the doorway of the hospital room. The third day, he walked into the hallway and to the nurse's station. On the fourth day, he walked around the entire floor. On the fifth day, he walked around the floor a few times and climbed some stairs. On the sixth day, he could walk around the floor, climb stairs, and get himself dressed. On the seventh day, Tim went home.

Every night, Tim increased his time walking on the treadmill. After a month, he could jog a mile, which he hadn't done since he was twelve. After four and a half months, Beth had a four-mile charity run for the CF Foundation that Tim took part in and completed. Being a personal trainer for twenty years was obviously an advantage for Tim, as he admits that at no point was the training painful.

By April, Tim was confident that he could run the race. So, he called Dr. Sonett to let him know that he'd be ready to go by November. By summer, Tim was already up to thirteen miles on his treadmill.

Tim trained and trained, but didn't see much of his surgeon. Dr. Sonett gave them a meeting point on race day. They met up, and Dr. Sonett had two shirts in his hand. One said "Lung transplant patient Tim" and the other said "Lung transplant surgeon" but no name. Tim asked why Dr. Sonett didn't put his name on there. His reply was, "I want people to cheer for you."

Tim and Dr. Sonett ran the entire race together. Tim managed to get through some cramping at the eighteen-mile mark by taking some electrolytes, but at no point did he feel that he was in jeopardy of stopping.

During the marathon, Tim had the unique privilege to have a six-hour conversation with Dr. Sonnet. "During that time, I asked him some important questions I had on my mind, like if he was emotionally connected with his patients at the time of surgery, or if it's easier to set his emotions aside so it wouldn't impact his performance. He told me that he is extremely invested in each and every one of his patients, and that is exactly how he is able to get his best performance. I still think about that today, as I think it is remarkable."

Still, it was the conversation at mile nine that stands out for Tim. "I asked him how much longer I had to live, a question I always had but was afraid to ask while living in the hospital. He said, 'About two weeks.' Here I was, running in the biggest marathon in the world next to the man who had saved me. I knew I would be okay no matter what his answer was going to be. I think about this moment every few days—way more memorable than crossing the finish line."

Tim asked if Dr. Sonett was going to let Tim win. Dr. Sonett said, "No, let's cross together." And so they did, interlocked hands raised in the air.

Tim says that looking back, the motivation he felt in 2010 came from knowing that if he could run a marathon less than a year out from a double-lung transplant, then not only could he do anything, he could also literally say, "I escaped death." He also understands that without a supportive family, countless nurses, PAs, specialists, and other volunteers who lent a hand, there is no way he would be alive today, much less a victor in the New York City Marathon.

Tim has since returned to his job as a personal trainer. His lifelong commitment to a good diet and exercise ensured his speedy recovery. He keeps in constant contact with Dr. Sonett. At one point, they considered writing a book together. He still admires the man who helped save his life.

"I am still in awe almost ten years later at the skill of someone who can literally save someone's life with their own hands. He is an incredible human being who goes around saving people almost every day. I call him the everyday Superman."

AARON HEROUX

Age: 42

Resides: New York, United States

Age at diagnosis: 18 months

Double-lung-transplant recipient; had a law passed in his honor in the state of New York allowing him the opportunity to apply for a job in law enforcement after the age of thirty-five; successfully passed the police-entry physical exam post-transplant at the age of forty; current sheriff deputy of Clinton County, New York

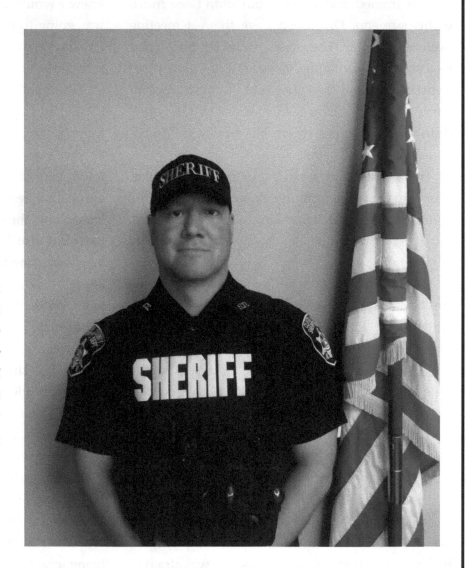

"With growing advancements in medicine, there will be more people like me that want to return to work [after] being told 'no.' and finally, there is hope for their return!"

Clinton County Sheriff Deputy Aaron Heroux has been enforcing the law for years, but it's one law in particular that he is proudest to defend.

Aaron was diagnosed in 1977 at eighteen months old, when cystic fibrosis was even less known than it is now. "I remember that the enzymes didn't come in capsules [at that time], so my mother made applesauce to mix with the granular enzyme," says Aaron. "Growing up, I stayed as normal as possible. The disease really wasn't that bad for me. I was able to play sports and move about whenever I wanted. My mother was the best. She never sheltered me or babied me. She would let me go outside and play, no matter how cold or how much I coughed. She told my grandmother once when I was outside in the winter, 'I don't know how long we have with him. I will not hold him back from doing what makes him happy.' Back in the eighties, I wasn't given much hope for the future. [The doctor] thought I would be dead at twelve. When I turned twelve, I was told eighteen. As I got older, the age just increased, so needless to say I never really planned for the future."

Aaron did not even have his first hospitalization until he was twenty, as his symptoms were extremely mild. He was pancreatic insufficient, with which the enzymes helped immensely, and though he had the incessant coughing, he had a nebulizer to inhale aerosols. He also had a ramp that his dad had built so that his parents would have an incline to more easily help Aaron perform postural drainage. His mild symptoms, his conventional and unconventional treatments, and his supportive parents added up to Aaron being able to participate in sports at the same level as his peers.

After being denied entry to the military because of his CF, Aaron went to college and earned an associate's degree in criminal justice. At twenty-three, he started working as a corrections officer at the Clinton County Sheriff's Office, and became a deputy sheriff in 2002. Aaron never hid the fact that he had cystic fibrosis, but he never used it as an excuse to get out of work or to acquire an easier post. He wanted to be treated like every other law-enforcement officer. Plus, he had the fortunate circumstance of his hiring manager, Sheriff Lawliss, having a granddaughter with CF, though he is not sure if Sheriff Lawliss even knew that Aaron had CF when he hired him.

Aaron says the first time he was ever afraid of his disease was during an episode on Christmas Day 2006, when he was thirty. "I was having an asthma attack," he says, "and could not take deep breaths. I was brought to the ER by my wife. Turned out I had an empyema, which is rare, and it basically fills the pleural lining of the lungs, causing pain with every breath, and grows bigger as time goes on. I had it for a month and couldn't figure out what was wrong with me. I permanently lost about ten percent of my lung function in that one incident."

But what is more memorable for Aaron about that event was the poise shown by his wife, Victoria. "I am married to a wonderful wife," he says. "She has been my rock in times that I truly needed someone. I didn't realize how much until I couldn't breathe."

Aaron's successful service as deputy came to an end after eleven years, when he had to go on disability retirement due to his deteriorating lung function. By that time, he was on oxygen 24/7. At one point, he was on twenty to twenty-five liters of oxygen on a high-flow machine. After a month's hospitalization in Boston and a nearly two-year wait, the doctors came to Aaron and asked if he was ready for new lungs. Aaron called Victoria, his brother, and his parents. "Being wheeled to the operating room," he says, "was the only time I was nervous for the procedure. I prayed that if something happens to me that my wife would be okay."

On February 8, 2014, Aaron received a double-lung transplant at Mass General Hospital in Boston. His doctors prepared him and Victoria that it may require a one- or two-month hospital recovery, but again praising his wife's support, Aaron was out of the hospital in ten days. He stayed in Boston for the next two months for follow-up tests, but suffered very few complications. He says he had some anxiety from the meds and that there was some concern about his heart function, but eventually he was good to go.

In May of 2014, just three months after his transplant, Aaron returned as a police dispatcher at the Clinton County Sheriff's Office. By July, he felt physically and mentally prepared to transition

back. Sadly, Aaron was told that at thirty-eight, he was too old and had been out of the position too long to return to his old post.

"I was surprised and could not understand or accept that my police career was over," he says. "For the next year and a half, each week I would meet with the current Clinton County sheriff, David Favro. We would research and reach out to different agencies, NYS Civil Service, and politicians. But, the Civil Service law was clear. It states that if you are over the age of thirty-seven and have been out of your position for over a year, you cannot return to service."

With the support of his wife, Victoria, and his best friend, Bill, Aaron took a stand. In December of 2015, Sheriff Favro was able to get a meeting with local State Representative Janet Duprey. "She stated that there was nothing in the New York State law that would allow me to return to service," he says, "so she was going to write a bill to make a new law and attempt to get it passed through the House and the Senate."

Representative Duprey held true to her promise. In June of 2016, the bill was passed by the House and Senate, and in July 2016, Governor Cuomo signed Bill A10226 and S07564 into law, which allowed Aaron to have an opportunity to retain his old job.

However, Aaron was not out of the woods yet. The day before his start date, he was told he had one year to pass an agility test. The test was divided into three parts that had to be completed with only minor breaks in between: twenty-nine sit-ups in a minute, eighteen push-ups without stopping, and a mile-and-a-half run in a little over thirteen minutes. He began training with his friend Bill, who had known Aaron since 2007 when he was hired as a deputy sheriff. Aaron says Bill, who had a US Marine background, is a straight shooter who does not deal well with excuses.

Though the goals felt within reach, Aaron found himself failing the tests repeatedly. After months of training with Bill, he knew it was more than a physical issue. "I would have panic attacks while running during the [practice] exam," he says. So, with only a few months left, he saw his doctors and a psychologist to help him with his anxiety. He also hired Mary, a triathlon trainer who trained him six days a week and taught him how to breathe and relax while running. Bill continued to encourage his friend. Eventually, everything came together. With only two days left to the expiration of the bill, after forty-one failed attempts, Deputy Heroux completed the run with nine seconds to spare.

Aaron says he could not have done this without Victoria, who constantly encouraged him, and of course Bill. "I only hope to be as good a friend to him as he has been to me."

Aaron's proud of the bill that bears his name, and says that the law is bigger than just him. "With the growing advancement in the field of medicine," says Aaron, "there will be more people like me that want to return to work [after] being told 'no,' and finally, there is hope for their return!"

JILLIAN MC NULTY

Age: 43

Resides: Longford, Leinster, Ireland

Age at diagnosis: Birth

2012 Dublin Marathon finisher; headed a two-year campaign to get government approval for Orkambi in Ireland; crowned Longford's All-Time Great in February 2019

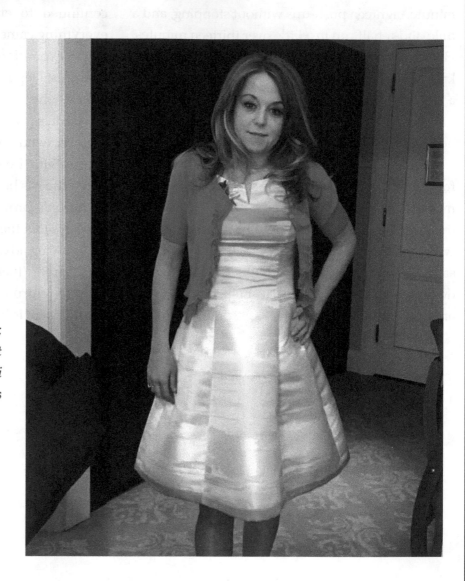

"I'd seen the miracle that was Orkambi so I wanted to fight for access for all people with CF eligible in Ireland."

Jillian Mc Nulty is extremely passionate about helping others with CF. She campaigns for the rights of people with CF, and has been actively campaigning in Ireland, the country with the highest per capita for cystic fibrosis in the world, for just over a decade. She was one of many campaigners who advocated for a dedicated unit for CF in St. Vincent's Hospital. Conditions were atrocious. "Conditions were so bad, CF patients had to share a six-bedded ward with other sick patients with the flu, pneumonia, etc. Toilets and showers were shared between the whole ward, which was used by thirty-two patients."

After years of campaigning, a six-story building went up in St. Vincent's. Now there are two dedicated CF floors, one outpatient and one inpatient, with twenty single rooms for CF patients.

Jillian's personal drive is more than just about social welfare, or even her own CF. "My parents have already had to bury two children—one with cystic fibrosis and one with special needs," she says, "and I don't want them to have to bury another."

In 2012, Jillian had remarkably trained in the hospital for three of the five months prior to running the Dublin Marathon with only 58 percent lung function, which would plummet after she was able to somehow complete the race.

"I stopped responding to IVs," Jillian says. "Months on them didn't bring my lung function back up, so then came Orkambi."

Jillian is referring to an FDA-approved "breakthrough therapy" drug for CF patients in the US that was part of a CF drug trial in Ireland. "I happened to be in the hospital when the research nurse asked if I wanted to take part. Obviously, I said yes, but she warned that I needed to be hospital- and IV-free for thirty days, and we didn't think I could last that long, as my admissions were every three to four weeks, five at a stretch. I somehow managed to stay out for four weeks and ended up in the hospital a few days after rigorous tests to go forward. It was so close. My PFTs had to be between forty and ninety percent to get through. I scraped through miraculously, getting forty-one percent. When I was told I got through, I cried my eyes out. This was hope for me. My CF had been in a very sharp decline the eight months previous.

"Seems strange, but before Orkambi, even though I was running, I was constantly exhausted, needed to take daily naps for hours to even function. A few months after I started taking Orkambi, I gradually started to feel normal again, and after a few years on it, my whole life was transformed. In the four and a half years I was on it, I no longer needed to nap—ever! My hospital stays previously were nine months of the year. In 2017, I had just one admission, in 2016, just three, and in 2015, no admissions, so I'd seen the miracle that was Orkambi. So, I wanted to fight for access for all people with CF eligible in Ireland."

Beginning in 2015, Jillian began a two-year

campaign for government approval of Orkambi in Ireland. That same year, Jillian was the only patient chosen outside of the US to fly to Washington, DC, to testify to the FDA approval committee for Orkambi.

Late in 2016, talks between the Health Service Executive (HSE), National Centre for Pharmacoeconomics (NCPE), and Vertex ended, and it was decided that Orkambi would not be made available to patients due to cost. Jillian organized a protest to take place at the government buildings on December 5, 2016, and thousands turned up in support, including senators. The following day, the HSE, NCPE, and Vertex announced they would reopen negotiations. The meeting took place on Thursday, January 5, 2017, and Orkambi was approved, as well as another life-saving CF drug, Kalydeco, which would become available for purchase in Ireland on April 11, 2017. Jillian's massive effort has made her a hero amongst her CF peers.

Does Jillian see herself as a hero? "I don't consider I have status as such. I'm just Jillian fighting for rights of CF patients. It's kind of surreal to think [of those days when] I was in full-time campaign mode. My days were sixteen to eighteen hours long. The work that went into organizing the protests was unreal. Now, getting messages from other patients and parents of those who've started [Orkambi] that their lives are changing is just so emotional. It makes it all worthwhile."

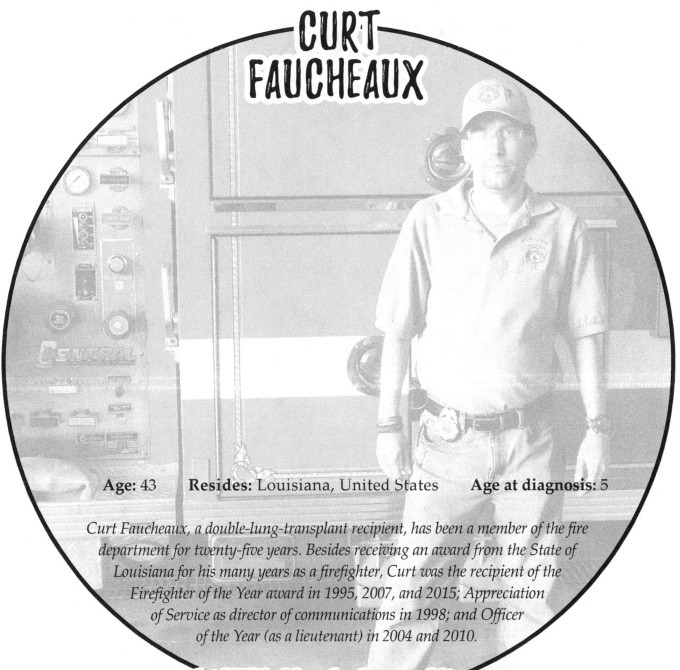

CURT
FAUCHEAUX

Age: 43   **Resides:** Louisiana, United States   **Age at diagnosis:** 5

Curt Faucheaux, a double-lung-transplant recipient, has been a member of the fire department for twenty-five years. Besides receiving an award from the State of Louisiana for his many years as a firefighter, Curt was the recipient of the Firefighter of the Year award in 1995, 2007, and 2015; Appreciation of Service as director of communications in 1998; and Officer of the Year (as a lieutenant) in 2004 and 2010.

"I never let [CF] hold me back or used it as a crutch. Instead, I used it to fuel my fire, so to speak, and prove the naysayers wrong."

NICHOLAS "NICK" TALBOT

Age: 43

Resides: London, England, United Kingdom

Age at diagnosis: 13

Current chief executive officer of International Valuation Standards Council (IVSC), a not-for-profit organization formed to strengthen the worldwide valuation profession in the public's interest

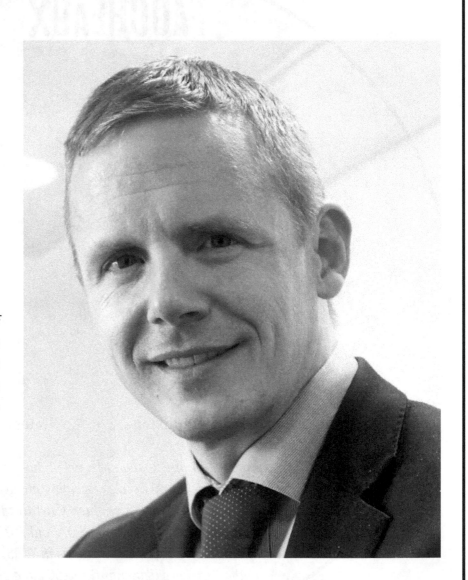

"I am not afraid of failure. If you don't fail at anything in life, you aren't pushing yourself and your limits."

Attempting to climb Mount Everest, the tallest mountain above sea level in the world at 8,848 meters, is a goal of many, but accomplished by few. Approximately three hundred people have died trying to achieve this feat. For anyone to say they've climbed Everest is incredible, but for a person with cystic fibrosis to do it, well, that's considered impossible. Meet Nick Talbot.

Nick grew up in the countryside of the United Kingdom, where the only thing a person could do was outside sports. His passions in life became skiing, traveling, spending time with friends and family, and his work. Nick runs an international not-for-profit organization trying to improve key parts of the global financial system for the benefit of everyone. He is famous, though, for his mountaineering, as he has climbed some of the tallest mountains in the world.

Nick remembers his introduction to the reality of CF. "I was admitted to the hospital in October of 1989 with three types of pneumonia," he says. "The only positive from my point of view was having a few months off from going to school! I was diagnosed with CF at the age of thirteen, and my parents were told they should expect I had about five years to live, though I only found this out last year! Rather than wrap me in cotton wool whilst I was still recovering, they went out and bought me a Christmas present, which was a mountain bike!"

Nick's fortunes turned with his introduction to Kalydeco. "I was lucky, as I have benefitted from life-changing drugs which only help five percent of us," he says. "Kalydeco improved my lung function about seven percent, but what I really noticed was how it cleared out my lungs completely in terms of coughing, and my times running certain distances kept improving over a two-month span." Nick was a part of various drug trials to help others battling cystic fibrosis.

Nick's training leading up to a big climb starts about six months prior. He runs up and down hundreds of flights of stairs, as well as a local hill, with ankle weights and an expedition rucksack of about sixty pounds. He does this for many hours, stopping only briefly for a small snack or an energy drink. On occasion he goes to the Alps to train, in which he carries his skis up the mountain and then skis back down before anyone else is there. "The training is mind-numbing and ridiculously hard, as I am constantly out of breath and trying to improve on my times."

Nick does his climbs to benefit the CF Trust, and has now climbed numerous mountains. However, he aspires to do something more. "I am trying to be the first person with cystic fibrosis to climb *the* Seven Summits (the highest summit on each continent), including Denali in Alaska and Vinson in Antarctica, to raise money and awareness for different CF charities. I think if all of us make a small effort, we will achieve more breakthroughs faster," he says. "The more people who do [make efforts], the more I believe will contribute money, and we know it is mainly down to the CF charities to fund new research."

To date, Nick has raised £120,000 directly for the CF Trust through his mountaineering. Indirectly, he raises more money by giving speeches at conferences and corporate events for local charities. Typically, a corporate speech will raise a five-figure sum of money for the local charity. Nick has spoken at some unusual venues, including Citifields Stadium, the University of Cambridge, and halfway up Mont Blanc.

It was in 2014, however, that Nick decided to do the ultimate climb. He decided it was time to try Everest. During any climb, Nick has a treatment routine that ensures he will keep his CF at bay while still accomplishing his goal. He brings his Kalydeco and some supplemental oral drugs for potential stomach issues. Before Kalydeco, he had to develop a different coughing technique to cope with the altitude. On one mountain, he tore the muscle down the side of his lungs from coughing. Pre-Kalydeco, he also used to lose a lot more weight during his climbs. In 2014, on Nick's first attempt, the mountain was closed after an avalanche killed a group of Sherpas in the icefall.

Undeterred, Nick tried again the following year and made it up to base camp. He was resting when "I felt scared, and what I saw was illogical. I got out of my tent to see a three-hundred-yard high wall of snow and ice coming toward me at about two hundred miles per hour," he says. An earthquake had shaken a large piece of glacier off the mountain, which crashed to the ground and took out the middle of base camp. Nick figures he had about ten seconds to react.

"My main concern was drowning. There were ice, rocks, gas canisters, ice axes, and other equipment flying through the air as the center of camp was spread over five hundred meters. A teammate, who was only a few meters away, unfortunately didn't make it. I was smashed into the ground, got up, and was smashed into the ground again. I was covered in cuts and blood, had a broken thumb, and a combination of broken and cracked ribs pressing into my right lung."

Nick displayed signs of hypothermia. He and his team were eventually able to stabilize his temperature by finding and then covering him with multiple sleeping bags. Nick and a few others were able to move down to a lower base camp, where he saw doctors who forced Nick to cough to avoid getting fluid and pneumonia in his right lung. Fortunately, the next day, helicopters were able to touch down and help Nick and his injured teammates.

Nick almost gave up on his dream to climb Everest because his mother was upset not knowing what happened to him in both big disasters, and his dad said he didn't want to see her crying again. "In the end, I decided to return because it was a choice of living life as I wished to, or as others wanted me to. My mother understood."

On Friday, May 13, 2016, in his third attempt,

after climbing for five days and dealing with a storm and oxygen failure, Nick accomplished something that no other CF patient had ever done: he "stood on top of the world." Nick Talbot had climbed Everest.

"When I finally hit the summit, I felt happy, emotional, relieved to have finally made it, and amazed to be up there, just myself and a Sherpa friend for fifteen minutes before the rest of the team joined us for another fifteen minutes. It felt a bit surreal to have finally done it, and even now it still feels a bit unbelievable."

Today, as one would expect, Nick looks back fondly on this amazing accomplishment. "Summiting Everest was one of the best days of my life. Looking back at it, it was a bit of a crazy challenge to take on, but a lot of good has come out of it in terms of profile and fundraising for CF charities."

In June of 2018, Nick continued his mountaineering adventures by becoming the first person with cystic fibrosis to climb Alaska's Denali, home of North America's tallest peak at 20,310 feet.

The secret of Nick's success is simple. "I am not afraid of failure. If you don't fail at anything in life, you aren't pushing yourself and your limits." Wise words from a man who accomplished the impossible.

ISABEL STENZEL BYRNES

Age: 47

Resides: California, United States

Age at diagnosis: Birth

Double-lung-transplant recipient; wrote the award-winning memoir along with her sister, Ana, called The Power of Two; *competed in the 2014, 2016, and 2018 Transplant Games of America and the 2017 World Transplant Games, where she amassed around forty medals*

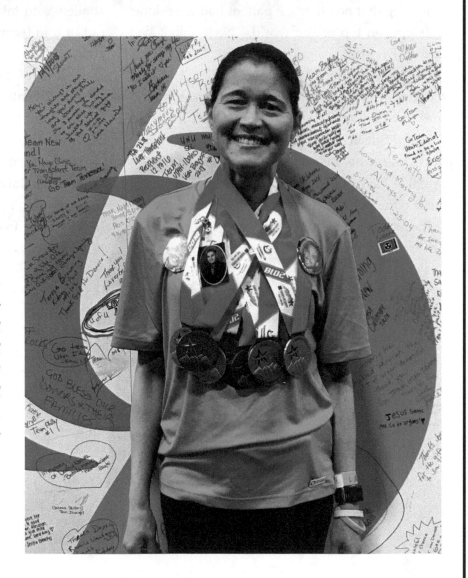

"To come to the edge of death and then to be reborn instills powerful emotions that are difficult to describe."

sabel and Ana, better known as the Stenzel twins, were born in the early seventies to a Japanese mother and German father. "My mother used to say that 'luck and misfortune are woven together like a rope,'" says Isabel, "and she could not have been more accurate. My sister, Ana, and I were born identical twins, and we were both born with cystic fibrosis."

At birth, their parents were told they would be lucky to reach age ten. So, from day one, Ana and Isabel traveled through life together, sharing the ups and downs of this terrible illness. Both twins dealt with the common CF symptoms: lung issues, stomachaches, and malabsorption, just to name a few. Isabel tells it this way: "We competed over who could tolerate longer treatments and who could even cough up more mucus to clear our lungs. When friends of ours with CF died, we held on tightly to each other, knowing that we were lucky we still had each other.

"Ana and I attended CF camp from age eleven to twenty-five. In addition to meeting our closest friends, we learned how to take care of ourselves, how to advocate for our health needs, and how to face the myriad of difficult emotions that CF brought on. We learned we weren't the only ones with this disease. We also learned that kids with CF die young, and some of our fate was up to our own discipline."

Isabel says that the risk of bacterial cross-contamination was far less important than the tremendous experience of meeting so many amazing people. She also said that the camps did have guidelines, and that campers were screened based on their sputum cultures. They were not allowed to cough on each other, share utensils, or do anything else that could lead to spreading germs.

"Ana and I acquired pseudomonas at the age of ten, and our adolescence was marked by regular cycles of pneumonia, as our bodies struggled to gain weight to go through puberty," says Isabel. "We each spent thirty-six weeks in the hospital by the time we reached eighteen, and used nighttime oxygen starting at age fourteen.

"Ana and I survived to graduate from high school, attended Stanford University, and each majored in human biology. We spent a year in Japan teaching English, manifesting our life philosophy that living fully was more important than living in a bubble. Plus, we had each other."

After Japan, the twins both attended graduate school at the University of California at Berkeley. Ana received a master's degree in genetic counseling; Isabel received a master's in public health and social welfare. They both got jobs at Lucile Packard Children's Hospital. The twins stayed close not just because of their love for one another, but also because they needed each other. They did each other's chest percussions, and that symbiotic bond kept them close and alive.

Shortly after starting her career, Ana's lungs deteriorated to the point that she was gasping for air. "In Ana, I saw what I would lose," said Isabel, "and I prepared for both of our deaths." Yet, thanks to a male organ donor, Ana received the gift of new lungs on June 14, 2000, at the age of twenty-eight.

Then, it was Isabel's turn. "Three years later, I found myself in Ana's shoes before her transplant," she says. "I had a massive lung bleed that left me oxygen dependent. After two years, at thirty-two, I slipped somewhat suddenly into lung failure, and was placed on a ventilator for twenty-three hours. Ana stood by my bedside, devastated and convinced she would soon be twin-less. Then, at the eleventh hour, on February 6, 2004, donor lungs were found."

In the following years, Ana and Isabel enjoyed energy they'd never experienced before. Their healthy lungs allowed them to swim competitively, run, hike places like Half Dome in Yosemite National Park and the Grand Canyon, and travel the world. Isabel herself followed her transplant by running two half marathons, swimming two thousand meters twice a week, and cycling twenty miles once a week.

"To come to the edge of death and then to be reborn instills powerful emotions that are difficult to describe," says Isabel. "The closest comparison would be falling madly in love. And so [Ana and I] both were—madly in love with life itself."

In 2007, Ana and Isabel continued their comeback by writing their memoir together called *The Power of Two: A Twin Triumph over Cystic Fibrosis* to chronicle their bond and their survival, and to express gratitude to all the medical advancements that made their achievements possible. The book was released just after Ana's second lung transplant in 2007 following a six-month bout of acute rejection. The twins traveled around the country to speak to the public, students, healthcare professionals, and CF families. They even visited Japan to speak about organ donation, a highly controversial subject there due to restrictive laws and religious reasons. "Without shame or hesitation, we went against convention and spoke openly about our illness journey," says Isabel, "what we had learned, and what we could teach others."

Their memoir inspired a documentary film called *The Power of Two*, released in 2011 at the prestigious DocuWeeks theatrical showcase in Los Angeles and New York City. The film received over ten awards and was featured in nearly forty film festivals. Isabel fondly looks back, "Our goal was simply to share our story—and hope it could be a vehicle to inspire others to cherish breath, to learn about cystic fibrosis, and to sign up to be organ donors. We hoped our message to others with illness would be clear—that sometimes illness is an opportunity for unconventional blessings. It has been a privilege to overcome CF, to become an illness ambassador, and to use our story to remind people of what they are capable of."

Ana and Isabel were riding high when, suddenly, Ana was diagnosed with small-bowel cancer just weeks after the debut of the film in DocuWeeks. She fought her cancer valiantly for two years before her death in September of 2013. She was forty-one.

Isabel struggled for several years with a deep and dark grief from the death of her twin. "Losing Ana was like an amputation," she says. "I miss her every day, and I feel like I am missing part of my consciousness. However, I had forty-one years to prepare for her loss. And, I appreciate having the anticipatory grief process, which allowed me to say and do everything I needed to with Ana before she left. I miss Ana on my birthday because it feels strange to grow older without her. I know she would be happy that I'm thriving, but it seems unfair that I get to live while she doesn't. I think of her whenever I experience profound moments of beauty and joy, like when I reach an athletic accomplishment or when I travel to special places I scatter her ashes at every national park I go to."

Ana had lived four times longer than her prognosis at birth, was married in 2010, had worked as a genetic counselor for sixteen years, and died shortly after the second edition of their memoir was released. Isabel says that her sister felt complete.

Isabel herself continues to speak publicly about CF and screens *The Power of Two* regularly, interspersed with her regular job as a bereavement coordinator at Mission Hospice. "I continue to add goals to my bucket list—travel, triathlons, getting my license in social work, etc.," she says. "I still have GI issues, diabetes, atrial flutter, osteoporosis, and skin cancer, but I am not defined by my diagnoses. I am defined by the glorious and extraordinary life that I have both been gifted with as well as created on my own.

"My grief without Ana has been intense, but both my organ donor and my husband of twenty years, Andrew, have kept me going. I am keeping my promise to Ana to exercise regularly and continue to compete at the Transplant Games of America." Isabel has won multiple medals since Ana left while competing in the 2014, 2016, and 2018 Transplant Games of America and in 2017 at the World Transplant Games. She says of her forty or so medals that the one that means the most is the one where they engraved Ana's face on the medal.

"She will always be with me."

PETER OXFORD

Age: 48

Resides: Sydney, New South Wales, Australia

Age at diagnosis: 1

Creator of Australia's first national dance competition, Showcase National Dance Championships; recently received a letter from Her Majesty Queen Elizabeth II congratulating him on his achievements and also his awareness campaigns for CF

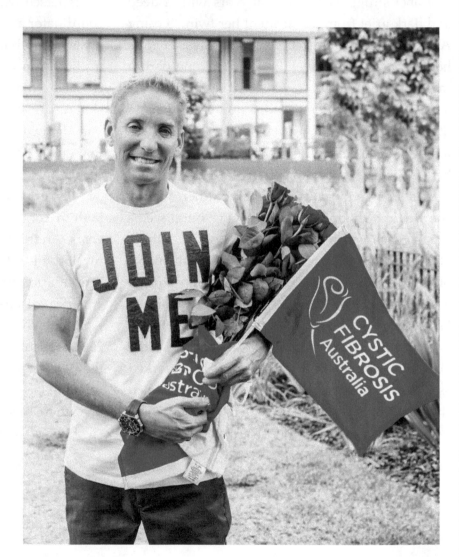

"I wouldn't be here now if I didn't dance."

As a youngster, Australian Peter Oxford—diagnosed with CF at one year old—met four other CF warriors while in the hospital, and they became a close-knit group. Back then, bacterial cross-contamination was not a known issue in the medical world, and CF patients were actually encouraged to spend time together. They made a pact that the lone survivor would "live their life for everyone."

At forty-eight, Peter is also one of the oldest Australians with cystic fibrosis. He finds himself a pretty big CF celebrity in Australia, as his national dance competition, Showcase National Dance Championships, which began with four hundred acts, now features more than eighteen thousand annually.

He was born in 1970 in Sydney, Australia, and one year later, upon diagnosis, his parents were told he was unlikely to reach his fifth birthday. Peter was interested in dancing, and began dance at the age of four primarily to help with his CF. It seemed to work, because he did not have a hospital admission until the age of fifteen. "I wouldn't be here now if I didn't dance. It keeps the airways clear the more exercise you can do." After the age of fifteen, though, his admissions became quite regular and were mostly sinus related.

Dance became his career and a sport that made him a celebrity. In July of 1993, Peter became the first Australian to win the American Dance Championships. Peter was also the first Australian to ever win back-to-back titles in Chicago, Orlando, and Las Vegas in the same year.

In 1994, Peter founded Australia's first nationally televised dance competition, Showcase National Dance Championships. After a quarter of a century, the show is recognized as the largest dance event in Australia's history, awarding over $2 million worth of cash and prizes over its twenty-four years, the largest amongst any other Australian dance competitions.

Despite the aid that dancing provided Peter's health, cystic fibrosis was never too far out of sight. Around the time he founded Showcase National Dance Championships, his four CF hospital mates each passed away from CF, all in their early twenties. "I am the last one of us, and that is something that I have always taken through my life," says Peter. "It's a very spiritual thing. I just know they're always around me." Peter also knows that it's important to keep his end of the deal and live his life for each of them.

Today, Peter spends much of his time inspiring the next CF generation. He recently spoke out about his own CF experiences during the National Cystic Fibrosis 65 Roses Campaign in Australia. He is an ambassador and peer-support leader for Cystic Fibrosis Australia.

Peter, who recently had a pneumothorax that required two drains and surgery to staple the lung, says, "CF has been part of my life. However, it lives with me. I don't live with it. Live your best life, I say, and turn dreams into reality, as they do come true."

This lone survivor kept his end of the deal.

BETH SUFIAN

Age: 53

Resides: Texas, United States

Age at diagnosis: 9

Attorney who concentrates on health law, has written two books, had over twenty articles published in medical journals, and presented more than one hundred speeches at hospitals and healthcare conferences; recipient of the Cystic Fibrosis Foundation's Alex Award; Time magazine recognized her as a "Local Hero" in 1996 for her service to people with disabilities

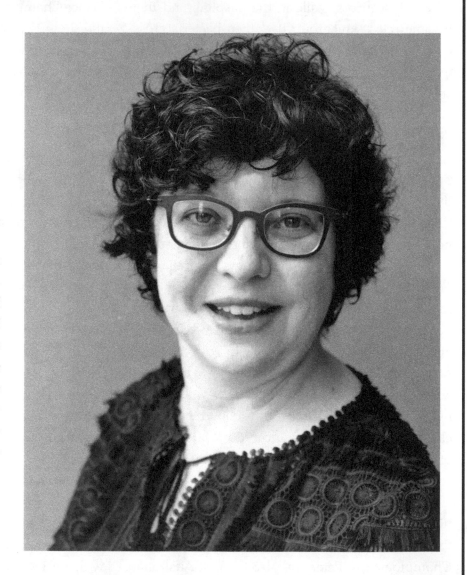

"I know how lucky I am and want to make sure I spend the time I have been given helping others."

Beth Sufian's path to becoming a zealous advocate for people with disabilities began at the University of Texas Law School. "My last year, I was in a children's rights clinic and represented a little girl who had lived in a hospital for five years. She had no family. I was just supposed to check in on her, but when I read through her file, I saw that a family had inquired about adopting her. The State had not followed up on the inquiry because the state caseworker had written, 'No one would want to adopt such a disabled child.' I contacted the family and worked for six months to make sure the girl could be adopted by the family. When she left the hospital to move to the West Coast, *Good Morning America* did a long story on her journey. Being involved with the case made me realize how important the law is to people with disabilities."

Beth was diagnosed with cystic fibrosis at nine years old, while her younger sister of two years was diagnosed at seven. She attended college at Emory University in Atlanta at a time when the only treatments for CF her doctor could prescribe were a drug called Mucomist®, which thinned secretions, and albuterol, which opened the airways. "I was lucky to be cared for at the Emory CF Center," she says. "The vest had not been developed, and so I went to the CF center every day for chest physical therapy. I was monitored by a wonderful physical therapist, Louis Batson, who kept a close watch on me. If he thought I was having even the slightest trouble breathing, he sent me up to see the amazing doctor, Dr. Daniel Caplan. These two men made it possible for me to finish college on time."

Among her college trials was becoming ill—suffering with a significant pulmonary exacerbation—on a Semester at Sea cruise ship her junior year. "I called my CF doctor, Dr. Glasser, from the middle of the Indian Ocean," says Beth, "and he called in a prescription for tobramycin, which I was using off label since TOBI was not available yet. I retrieved the medicine in Hong Kong, where my CF doctor was able to find a pharmacy, and felt better in just two days and was allowed to continue on the trip around the world." Beth says that had it not been for inhaled tobramycin, she does not believe that she would have lived past her thirties.

After law school, Beth went to work at a big law firm in Houston and found the perfect mentor in Collyn Peddie. "When she left to go work at a boutique litigation firm, I followed her. I handled a large number of cases that went to trial and perfected my litigation skills."

However, the dues she had to pay for a successful law career, let alone that of a litigator, wreaked havoc with her CF. "I worked eighty hours a week, and there was little time to rest or do the few breathing treatments that were available at the time," she says. "Thankfully, I was concurrently seeing CF physician Dr. Jack Jacoby, who was at the St. Vincent's CF Center in New York City. I started going to New York for care because my sister, who lived in New York, raved about Jacoby, her CF doctor."

The effort had never paid off more for Beth than at this professional and personal crossroads. "Dr. Jacoby helped me understand the importance of taking care of myself. When my health hit rock bottom from working too much, we had a heart-to-heart talk. He told me that the prestige of my job and the money I was making would mean nothing if I was no longer alive. I told him I had started helping people with CF in Houston who needed help with Social Security cases, and confided that perhaps I might start my own firm with a focus of helping people with CF. Dr. Jacoby encouraged this idea and told me I would make a tremendous difference in the lives of people with CF if I pursued this dream. He helped me see a different life path."

Beth left the law firm and started her own firm in 1994. After working at a loss for a few years, her husband of six years, James Passamano, joined the firm. The firm continued representing people in Social Security matters and helped companies trying to gain reimbursement from health-insurance companies, Medicaid, and Medicare.

In 1998, Beth started the CF Legal Information Hotline so that she could provide free and confidential legal information to people with CF. The hotline is now funded by a grant from the CF Foundation and, over seventy-two thousand calls later, continues to serve eight thousand callers a year. There is no other service that offers free and confidential information to people with CF from attorneys who have spent twenty-five years advocating for the cause.

In 1992, a physician at Texas Children's Hospital CF Center in Houston, Texas, asked if Beth could help a patient who had been trying to get SSI benefits for three years. The patient was scheduled for a hearing before a judge and could not find an attorney to help him. "I decided to help the child and learned as much as I could about Social Security benefits," she says. "We won the case, and the judge complimented me on my presentation, which gave me the confidence to take more cases. My CF center asked me to handle many more cases, and I agreed." Beth did not charge her clients because they were all low income and could not afford to pay.

For many years, Beth handled hundreds of cases for people with CF without charging a fee, and as word spread throughout the United States, she had a large number of people asking for help. Then, in 2010, Beth received funding to help twenty-five patients apply for Social Security benefits. "I was able to help people obtain benefits within thirty to ninety days of filing the application," she says. "The national waiting period is two to three years. I realized if I had funding to help people with an application for benefits, I could help them get the benefits quickly. This would allow people to have the money they needed to pay for housing and food, and obtain the insurance that comes with eligibility for benefits."

So, Beth started the CF Social Security Project

in 2011, which is also funded by a grant from the CF Foundation. Her firm has now successfully represented thousands of people in Social Security matters.

Beth feels fortunate to be as healthy as she is, and attributes it to her husband of thirty years, James, their eighteen-year-old daughter, Isabella, her parents and sisters, her medical team, and the CF pioneers who have taught her so much about managing her life and being a successful advocate.

Some of those CF trailblazers include Catherine Martinet, Pammie Post, Isabel Stenzel Byrnes, and Ana Stenzel.

"My life has been enriched by my relationships with people with CF," she says. "So many have come before me and shown me how to be strong and how to care about those who are less fortunate than myself. I know how lucky I am, and want to make sure I spend the time I have been given helping others."

PHIL WENRICH

Age: 56

Resides: Pennsylvania, United States

Age at diagnosis: Birth

Served on the board of directors and as the chairman of the national volunteer leadership initiative for the Cystic Fibrosis Foundation's Delaware Valley chapter; served on the board of the United States Adult Cystic Fibrosis Association; co-editor of the Society News *(a nonprofit newsletter serving the healthcare community); served as president and chairman of the Cystic Fibrosis Society*

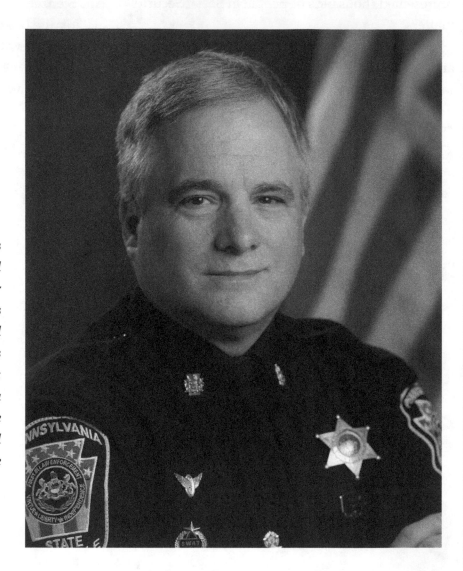

"I remember [my doctor] telling me that I would never be able to cope with such a demanding career, and his opinion became my motivation to make it happen."

In 1952, Phil Wenrich's parents, Bernard and Bettie, were among the original people who chartered the Cystic Fibrosis Association. In 1955, that association went on to become the Cystic Fibrosis Foundation, for which Phil became a poster child in 1971. The very first poster child, however, was Phil's brother, Bernie, who passed away from the disease at twelve years old, a year before Phil was born.

While Phil never met Bernie, his passing definitely affected his life. "My parents thought they were going to lose me at a young age, as well," he says. "So, there was always that fear there because they already lived this path. My father was tough on me and pushed me to live a normal life, and my mother coddled me and overnurtured me because she was afraid she was going to lose another son. From as young as I can remember, I used the latter motivation to fight as hard as I possibly could in the hope of finding a way to the former."

Phil's father was a police officer, which initially inclined Phil toward a career in law enforcement. Extra inspiration came in the form of a skeptical doctor. "I remember him telling me when I was around sixteen years old that I would never be able to cope with such a demanding career," he says, "and his opinion became my motivation to make it happen."

Phil started his police-and-public-safety career in 1985 at the age of twenty-two, when he graduated the police academy. Phil says he was fairly healthy at the time he attended the police academy, and therefore was able to blend in pretty easily, despite the long hours. His tenure at the academy was six months' worth of forty- to fifty-hour weeks of activity strenuous enough to make Phil suspect that CF would eventually catch up with him. "Although I pushed through all obstacles," he says, "it was still in the back of my mind, especially every time I had a CF flare-up."

He remembers his first really big CF scare at the age of twenty-three. "I was standing in a stairway waiting for my partner and coughed up blood for the first time," he says. "I was scared to death."

The majority of Phil's coworkers were unaware of his CF for most of his career. However, even though the ones who did know didn't discuss it, he admits the job was challenging. "There are, unfortunately, physical altercations that require a whole lot of lung capacity to breathe your way through. I remember a specific incident when a guy sexually assaulted a woman, and we had to handcuff him and carry him about a hundred yards to the police car because he would not cooperate and was continuing to fight," he says. "That was the first time that I was really struggling to breathe."

Still, Phil's passion has guided him through a variety of demanding but fulfilling jobs over the past thirty-four years. He has served as a police motorcycle officer, narcotics detective, assistant state police fire marshal, an emergency management coordinator, road master, and fire marshal for his local municipality. Today, Phil continues his law-enforcement career as a Pennsylvania State constable. He is a nationally registered emergency medical technician and state-certified EMS instructor. Phil, who himself attained the rank of black belt in martial arts, also served as an official and coach of the National Amateur Athletic Union coaching martial-arts competitors.

Phil can definitely look back at a number of accolades that have come his way while serving in law enforcement. He has been honored for lifetime achievements by elected officials. He received a personal note from President George W. Bush congratulating him on the honor, and official citations from the US Senate, US House of Representatives, US Congress, the Pennsylvania Office of the Governor, the Pennsylvania Senate, and the Pennsylvania House of Representatives soon followed. To top it all off, a flag was flown over the United States Capitol building in Phil's honor.

Life was great for Phil, but CF eventually started taking its toll. "The years had gotten tougher and tougher," says Phil. "I continued to do most of the things I had always done, like being an avid motorcycle rider and instructor, but the effort had become monumental and downright crippling."

Phil says he had to keep "upping his game," which basically meant exercising, going out with family, and doing all the things that normal people did, but with very little energy. "When I got to the point of all my strength exhausted, I simply got stronger and attacked it over and over again. I can look back and say cystic fibrosis stopped me from doing absolutely nothing that I wanted to do."

Despite his resolve, Phil found himself in end-stage CF, awaiting lung transplant. "I focused on my wife, Lisa, and our young son, Liam," says Phil. "They got me to tomorrow."

On September 27, 2017, at fifty-four years of age and after numerous false alarms, Phil had a successful double-lung transplant. For the first time in years, he feels like he can breathe again. Although eternally grateful to his donor and their family, the transplant process and recovery have not been without challenges, such as rejection, the flu, and cytomegalovirus (CMV). "My lungs changed, but not my fighter's mentality. My mindset has always been bulletproof. No matter what comes my way, I just roll right through it."

Phil says, "I appreciate the little things in life that most take for granted, like walking their dog, going to the market, and taking walks on the boardwalk with my family. Tomorrow is not guaranteed to anyone. Live for today."

TIM WOTTON

Age: 48   **Resides:** London, England, United Kingdom   **Age at diagnosis:** 6 months

*Reaching forty in 2011 was such a dramatic, life-affirming landmark for Tim Wotton
that this husband, father, and former junior international field-hockey player
decided to share his experiences and survival lessons in order to help others.
Tim has increased CF publicity in the UK and globally by opening up
through his* Postcards from Earth *blog, his award-winning
CF memoir* How Have I Cheated Death?, *and
engaging in public speaking.*

"Actually 'wanting to' rather than 'having to' be healthy is very empowering."

JERRY CAHILL

Age: 62

Resides: New York, United States

Age at diagnosis: 11

Graduated cum laude from the University of Connecticut; New York City Marathon finisher in 1991 and 1993; skin cancer survivor; motivational speaker and author; inspiration behind the "You Cannot Fail" merchandise line provided by the Boomer Esiason Foundation; developed the Team Boomer program and Exercise for Life scholarship for CF student athletes; subject of the award-winning documentary Up for Air

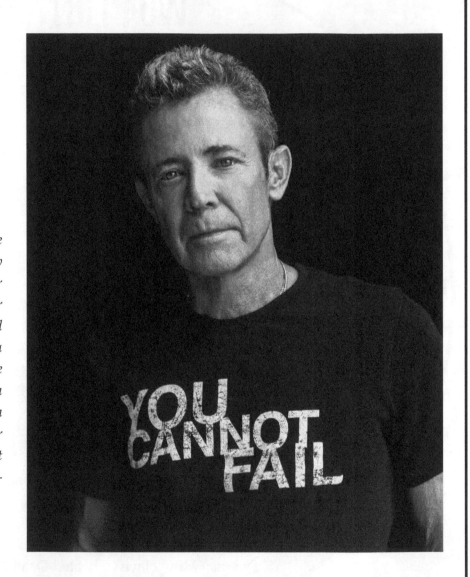

"Everybody has things in life they have to overcome, and you just have to believe you cannot fail."

Three months after having his lung transplant, when many transplant patients are still convalescing in the hospital, Jerry Cahill crossed the finish line of the Boomer's Cystic Fibrosis Run to Breathe, a 10K in New York City's Central Park. He not only finished the race, but did so with Joshua Sonett, MD, the surgeon who performed the procedure, running right beside him—the same Dr. Sonett who transplanted and ran the New York City Marathon with fellow CF warrior Tim Sweeney. Jerry finished the race in ninety minutes, actually exceeding his time from the previous year.

For the first eleven years of his life, Jerry was weighed down by a chronic cough, exhaustion, and the inability to gain weight. When he was finally diagnosed with CF at age eleven, doctors told his parents, Edward and Mary, that he'd be fortunate to see his eighteenth birthday. Edward wouldn't stand for this negative prognosis, nor would Jerry's three older brothers, all athletes.

Jerry was encouraged to play various sports including baseball, basketball, and football. In high school, he found a passion for track and field, specifically pole vaulting. He loved that it required gymnastics, running, weight-lifting skills, and most of all, the existential challenge of man against bar. His record pole vault in high school was 12'6".

Leaving the worry over his life expectancy in the dust, Jerry was healthy enough to compete in pole vaulting collegiately at the University of Connecticut, where he eclipsed 14'3", and later at the New York Athletic Club, where he won several awards with a 16'3" vault. This was only a few feet short of qualifying for the Olympics. Jerry went on to eventually compete in master's competitions. He peaked at number four in the nation with USA Track & Field (USATF). "I wasn't concerned with being the first person with CF to do anything. I was just competing against me."

Jerry, a member of the Catholic High School Athletic Association Hall of Fame, actively participated in pole vaulting into his midfifties. While lung complications from CF curbed his competition career, he discovered a new purpose for his athletic pursuits. He found that exercising, specifically running, helped him to loosen the mucus in his lungs. For a handful of years, while Jerry was in his fifties, doctors wanted to activate him on the lung-transplant list, but believing he was deriving enough lung power from exercise, he asked them to delay it as long as possible. Eventually, he found that even a diligent exercise program wasn't sufficient, and about a year after doctors initiated the conversation, they told him it was time.

Months prior to his transplant, Jerry was still jogging with an oxygen tank and a lung function of 23 percent. Doctors finally found Jerry's match when Jerry's lung function dipped down to 19 percent.

Three months after having his successful lung transplant, he not only participated in, but had that remarkable showing at Boomer's Cystic Fibrosis Run to Breathe. Today, Jerry is an ambassador for the Boomer Esiason Foundation (BEF), heading up the BEF scholarship and transplant grant programs. He also records educational podcasts along with the CF Wind Sprint video series explaining the importance of exercise, whether performed in the mountains or on a hospital bed.

Jerry currently coaches pole vaulting at three high schools in the New York area. His mantra, "You cannot fail," gifted to him by his parents when he was young and suffering, is not just for fellow CF patients, but also the athletes he coaches. Jerry explains, "Everybody has things in life they have to overcome, and you just have to believe you cannot fail."

His passion for never giving up helped him write a children's book in 2013, *Jerry, the Boy Who Could Not Fail*. The mantra also inspired a clothing line and even a scholarship provided by the BEF granting $5,000 to one male and one female winner to the institution of their choice.

In September of 2018, Jerry and his good friend and fellow CF warrior Emily Schaller completed their fifth five-hundred-mile Bike to Breathe tour, an event which Jerry founded. His FEV1, which pretransplant was around 19 percent, now hovers between 104 percent and 108 percent.

The boy who could not fail hasn't.

LISA BENTLEY

Age: 49   **Resides:** Caledon, Ontario, Canada   **Age at diagnosis:** 20

Lisa has won eleven Ironman races and eleven Ironman 70.3 (1/2 Ironman) races. She also represented Canada on multiple national teams and at the Pan American Games, and was ranked top five in the world in the Ironman standings for a decade. In her retirement, she finished second amongst women over forty at the 2013 ING Marathon, and first amongst women over forty-five at the 2014 Boston Marathon. She was inducted into the Etobicoke Sports Hall of Fame in 2012 and to the Triathlon Canada Hall of Fame in 2014. In retirement, she has been running marathons, doing motivational speaking and television commentary, and recently published her first book, An Unlikely Champion. Learn more about Lisa's tremendous accomplishments at www.LisaBentley.com.

"CF is not a death sentence.
Rather, it is a reason to move and exercise and live full."

BARBARA M. HARISON

Age: 72

Resides: California, United States

Age at diagnosis: 64

Started the Loretta Morris Memorial Fund with the Cystic Fibrosis Lifestyle Foundation (CFLF) in 2010, which has awarded 157 recreation grants to children and adults living with cystic fibrosis

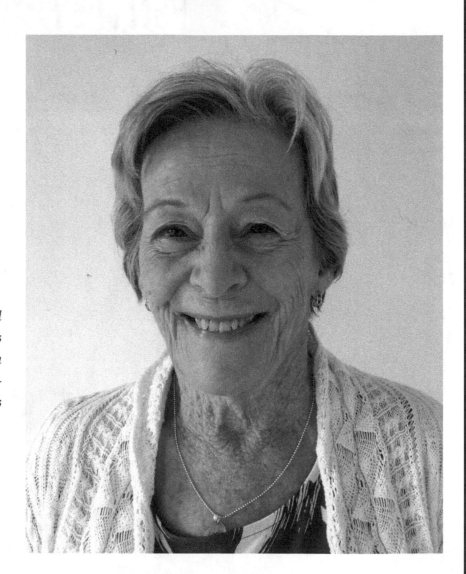

"I am healthier now in my seventies than when I was in my sixties!"

Not only is Barbara M. Harison one of the older CF fighters in the world, but she is also one of the latest diagnosed at the age of sixty-four.

As children growing up together, Barbara and her younger sister, Loretta, shared both a bedroom and respiratory problems. "We were both often sick, but she was usually sicker," says Barbara, who had scarlet fever when she was five. "My mom, a polio survivor, was frustrated with pediatricians that couldn't address my sister's health problems. Yet, she was persistent, and after years witnessing her daughter suffer, Loretta was finally diagnosed with CF when she was sixteen years old."

Barbara remembers losing Loretta, who passed away in 1971 at the young age of twenty-one. "That summer, she and I traveled in my 1969 VW Bug from San Francisco, California, to British Columbia, Canada. I didn't know it then, but it was to be our first and last trip together. I didn't realize how severely CF had affected my sister, as we were not living in the same household at that time. CF affected Loretta's lungs and pancreas. She was only five foot two and weighed eighty pounds. It was challenging on the trip for her to keep up with the treatments she needed. But, we wanted to take a vacation together, and Loretta did not want to give up, even when she was getting weak and sick.

"On the way back from Canada, I was worried that she needed to get to a hospital. I had to carry her baggage and equipment everywhere. I called my mom when we were overnight in a motel in Washington State. Mom said to get her on a plane home. The next day I got her booked on a flight from Portland, Oregon, to Los Angeles. It was a sad farewell and a lonely trip back home for me."

Loretta rallied one more time at UCLA Medical Center and went back to college, but died just two months after their trip on November 15, 1971. "I was sorry I could not get to Southern California before she died. I can remember flying down and crying the whole trip. Once I arrived, I helped my parents with the funeral services. I never saw my mother so sad and broken up. I think Loretta knew she did not have much time to live and was determined to travel, living on the edge, doing what she wanted to do. My parents did not hold her back."

Several years after Loretta died, Barbara's lung problems included bronchiectasis and pneumonia. "When I was in my early thirties, I went to Stanford Pediatric Center and was told I was likely a carrier with symptoms." In actuality, one in thirty-one people in the United States are carriers of CF, although there are some who have harsher symptoms despite not having the actual disease.

There wasn't genetic testing then and not much treatment was available, other than the manual percussion treatment known as postural drainage. Barbara's husband, Richard, assisted with this procedure for a while, but eventually Barbara decided exercise would serve her better than percussion.

"I had a busy career and adapted to reduced

lung capacity, and went on many years living well as long as I didn't catch a cold," she says. "As I headed into my fifties and sixties, I had more frequent pneumonia, shortness of breath, and coughing, though never hospitalized. I just got by with oral antibiotics. I was treated by several doctors who just didn't get that I could have CF, even when I told them my family history and symptoms. They just thought I was too old and that I had COPD or bronchiectasis. It was frustrating."

Finally, one doctor looked at the possibility that she could have CF.

In 2010, Dr. Richard Belkin at Santa Barbara Pulmonary Associates diagnosed Barbara with CF. "This was actually a blessing," she says, "as I now have the benefit of the latest CF treatments. It was a whole new regimen to undertake at age sixty-four, but all seemed to help ease the CF symptoms, and I could last longer at exercise and not get short of breath."

Being pancreatic sufficient, Barbara does not take enzymes. She also does not use the vest, as she says that her experience with it over the years did not provide her the airway clearance that many others received. Exercise, which she has been actively doing since the age of thirty, served that purpose. "My exercise regimen in lieu of the vest is swimming laps for forty minutes three times a week, walking two or more times a week for forty minutes or more, playing golf at least once a week, and doing some yoga or Pilates," she says.

Drawn to water and beaches all her life, she says she is fortunate to live on the Pacific Coast in Ventura, California, and get the added benefit of moist salt air on beach walks.

Barbara is now retired and believes in "giving back" through donations and volunteering. "This is how I connected with the Cystic Fibrosis Lifestyle Foundation (CFLF)," she says. "Its mission fit well with my own interests, and I could help others with CF through recreation grants to help them stay active and healthy."

In memory of her sister, Barbara started the Loretta Morris Memorial Fund with the CFLF in 2010. Since then, the fund has awarded 157 grants to children and adults living with CF. Barbara also served on the CFLF board for several years.

While CF can be a scary diagnosis, it allowed Barbara to make a plan to combat her previously unknown condition. She is now doing various aerosol treatments as well as taking antibiotics, multivitamins, and Kalydeco, which has resulted in improved lung function and a happier and more productive life. "The official diagnosis of CF led me to the treatment I needed," she says. "I am healthier now in my seventies than I was in my sixties!"

JAMES "JIM" DRESCH

Age: 77   **Resides:** South Dakota, United States   **Age at diagnosis:** 51

Jim, a father, grandfather, and great-grandfather about to celebrate his fiftieth wedding anniversary with his wife, Joan, not only has cystic fibrosis, but is also a diabetic and colon cancer survivor. He has owned the same hairstyling salon, Clipper Jim's, for more than forty-five years, and throws an annual golf tournament called The Clipper Jim Invitational. In its first seven years, the tournament has raised $430,000 for the Cystic Fibrosis Foundation, including a record $80,000 at the most recent event in 2018.

"The key to a successful life is accepting the hand each one of us is dealt while maintaining a positive attitude."

PAUL QUINTON

Age: 74

Resides: California, United States

Age at diagnosis: 19

Nancy Olmsted chair in pediatric pulmonology; professor of pediatrics at the University of California, San Diego (UCSD); discovered that the basic defect in the cystic fibrosis sweat duct was due to anion impermeability, which, to date, is considered a major breakthrough in understanding the basic CF defect

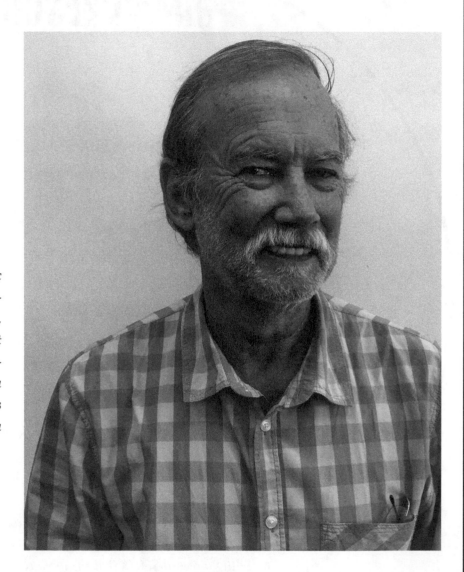

"The fact that I was more than twelve years older than the expected age for CF patients had little impact on my conclusion. I was convinced CF was my disease."

Dr. Paul Quinton considers science his religion, but he didn't always feel this way. It was one man who pointed the now seventy-four-year-old scientist in the direction of his career and changed—and maybe even saved—his life.

Paul was born in 1944, just six years after CF was recognized as a disease for the first time by Dr. Dorothy Andersen. Shortly after his first birthday, his mother told his pediatrician that he coughed a lot and couldn't get rid of colds. His pediatrician diagnosed him as having chronic bronchitis and said that Paul would just have to "live with it."

For the most part, having a chronic disease was a nuisance, and it was sometimes embarrassing for him to cough so much in public. The cystic fibrosis symptoms were definitely there. Paul sometimes felt lousy with chest pains, chills, and low-grade fevers, especially in the winters while he waited on the school playground to open. He was also rail thin and dealt with frequent stomachaches. Then, the big one that should have signaled to his physicians that Paul likely had CF: most of his shirts were stained from the high salt level in his sweat during the hot Texas summers—something he noticed was unique amongst the members of his family.

At sixteen, Paul was still coughing a lot, and the thought was that his upper right lobe could be the cause with its severe bronchiectasis and chronic-infection load. Being that this was a burden of chronic infection on his respiratory health, his upper right lobe was removed. "Removing it may have lightened the burden," he admits.

Paul was an inquisitive young man. Early in his second semester of his junior year at the University of Texas, he began studying the basis of his chronic cough, something the doctors diagnosed as bronchiectasis. He was curious as to how long people with bronchiectasis could expect to live. He pored through medical textbooks and, in one particular book, noticed a footnote: "See in connection with cystic fibrosis." Paul immediately combed the library to find information on CF.

Cystic fibrosis, which characterized many of his symptoms, was defined as a fatal disease, with patients not surviving beyond six to seven years of age. A cold chill ran down his back. While he was relieved to have finally solved the mystery, the overall outcome was perplexing. "Now, I read a death sentence—mine. I would soon die. The fact that I was already more than twelve years older than the expected age for CF patients had little impact on my conclusion. I read and reread the descriptions and matched them with mine. I was convinced CF was my disease."

After Paul told his doctor that he wanted to be tested for CF, his pulmonologist, Dr. Jenkins, sent him to Houston to see Dr. Gunyon Harrison, director of the first CF clinic in the Southwest. After three sequential sweat tests, Dr. Harrison confirmed Paul's self-diagnosis. He was the oldest CF patient Dr. Harrison had seen. Paul asked Dr. Harrison, "Well, how long am I going to live?"

Dr. Harrison had never seen a case like Paul's, so he simply responded, "Hell, I don't know."

Knowing how inquisitive Paul was, Dr. Harrison offered him a summer job in his CF clinic and laboratory. At the time, Paul was a premed and English major at the University of Texas. Paul wanted to know why pseudomonas aeruginosa was able to reside in the CF patients' lungs much more than in other lungs—a question that, forty years later, is just beginning to be answered.

By the end of the summer, Paul found out he had been admitted to medical school and ran into Dr. Harrison's office to tell him his good news.

"Are you crazy?" Dr. Harrison shouted. "You're going to pick up a bug in an emergency room, and you're going to be dead. You don't want to be a doctor. You want to be a scientist." Dr. Harrison sent him to Dr. Charles Philpott at Rice University to become a scientist. Four years later, Paul received his PhD in cell biology, skipping the master's program.

"Dr. Philpott knew I had CF, but I had resolved not to tell anyone I didn't absolutely have to about it. Among the people who fell under the 'need to know' category were my mentor on the student exchange I was on in Chile, my PhD advisor, and some very close friends that I thought it was important to be bare honest with."

Paul's reasons for secrecy were twofold. First, Paul understood that death was a difficult thing to deal with. He didn't want his presence to constantly remind people of that morbid subject, nor did *he* want to be reminded. Second, he wanted to make sure that whatever he was given was earned and not handed to him out of pity.

While working at the University of California, Riverside, Paul and his team analyzed the sweat ducts of CF patients. They discovered the abnormality in CF ducts was due to an impermeability to chloride. In other words, chloride ions could not get back across the duct cell membranes to be reabsorbed back into the blood, and therefore ended up in high concentrations on the surface of the skin. This conclusion explains the salt stains unique to CF patients' clothing, and was a key finding in the war against cystic fibrosis.

Through Paul's tireless lab work, he and his team also realized that bicarbonate, another anion like chloride, is also impermeable in CF, which helps explain why CF mucus is so abnormally thick and viscous. Further, Paul and his team have discovered how small airways in the lung are able to keep the surface of normal bronchiole tubes just wet enough to keep clean, but never too dry or flooded with fluid.

Paul is still doing well. At age fifty, he had his remaining upper lobe removed approximately thirty-four years after losing the right one. He still has occasional hospitalizations, which he playfully refers to as "jail." He credits Kalydeco, which he began taking in 2013, and Symdeco, which he began using in 2018, as two enormous reasons for his improved quality of life, and he is hopeful the entire CF community will have access to life-changing drugs like these in the future. He is now semiretired from working as a professor emeritus of pediatrics at the University of California, San Diego, where he continues to study the disease that ravages lungs.

And while he may owe his life to a doctor who told him to become a scientist, it's cystic fibrosis that may owe its death someday to Dr. Paul Quinton.

IN MEMORY

This book is about CF warriors, but unfortunately, not every warrior's journey continues after this book. I initially thought about not publishing Claire's, Natalie's, or Libby's stories because the goal of this book is to show young people with CF that they have plenty of time to accomplish their dreams. However, it occurred to me that even though these special women did not live to what most of us would consider middle age, one could make a strong case that they each achieved a tremendous amount. They deserve to be recognized.

CLAIRE WINELAND

Age at passing: 21

Resided: California, United States

Age at diagnosis: Birth

TEDx speaker; founder of Claire's Place Foundation, a 501(c)(3) not-for-profit organization, which has provided financial assistance of more than $1 million to over one hundred families; her YouTube channel has amassed more than 300,000 subscribers; worked on the set and was the inspiration behind the 2019 feature film Five Feet Apart

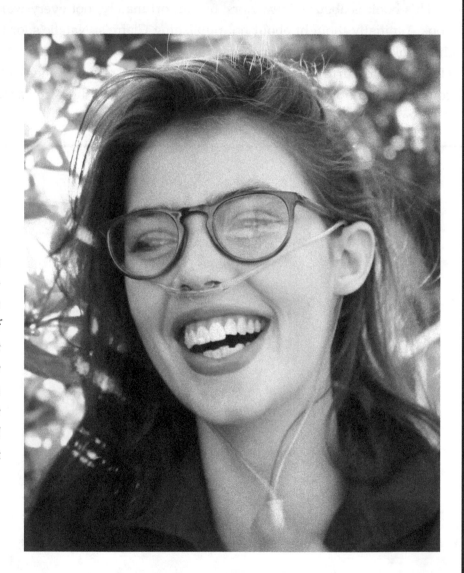

"The moment you let go of what you think your life should look like for you to be happy is the moment you actually start living."

Activist, entrepreneur, author, and TedX speaker Claire Wineland had to live a quarter of her life in the hospital—which included thirty surgeries—away from school, friends, and "normalcy." Yet, she attributed her success to the "joy and beauty and passion" she found through those hospital experiences.

"I had adventures through the hospital hallways and grew to love the doctors and nurses as if they were my family," she said. "This is because the moment you let go of what you think your life should look like for you to be happy is the moment you actually start living."

Claire's awareness not just of her disease but of her need for personal agency kicked in early. "I was around seven years old," she recalled, "and I was all alone in the hospital, feeling down on myself and separated from the rest of humanity. The doctors were talking over my head, and the nurse wasn't being friendly, and I felt lost. It was in that moment that I realized that if I wanted people to treat me with respect in the hospital, I had to earn it.

"So, I smartened up. I spent months learning every medication I was on, every procedure I had ever had. I learned how to 'speak doctor' and how to properly take care of myself. And more importantly, I learned how to warm up to strangers by developing this charming and funny persona that ensured people would see me as more than my illness.

"This changed my life completely, because all of a sudden I wasn't a victim of my situation. I had control over how people saw me and how people treated me. A few months later, I started decorating my hospital room and began feeling more at home in the hospital. I was in control of my own experience. No one could tell me how my life was going to play out. That was for me to decide."

Claire did not learn all this by herself. "I had an incredible support system growing up—not just parents and extended family, but nurses, nannies, and stepparents, as well. No one let me pity myself too much, and everyone had different tools to teach me on how to deal with my illness. For example, my father . . . taught me how to be a huge advocate for my own health and body, while my mom taught me how to be gentle with myself, and showed me that life is about more than just health—that I couldn't carry around guilt for not being the perfect patient all the time. I had a stepmom and nanny that taught me how to play games during treatments and make the whole thing fun."

So, with the help of such an amazing support system, Claire developed an extensive, disciplined treatment routine that she honed into a fine art. "I do around four to five hours of breathing treatments every day," she said, "which includes the vest, nebulized medications, and a boatload of coughing. I also take pills with every meal, around thirty-five in total. I take shots every night and hook up to a nightly feeding tube to squeeze in those extra calories. I have to eat around four thousand calories in a day, which is harder than it might seem, and get enough exercise to ensure that nothing gets too stuck in my lungs.

"Cystic fibrosis is an incredibly time- and energy-consuming disease, and it's easy to feel stuck in a never-ending cycle of treatments, pills, coughing, and more pills. You have to really love your life when you have CF, or else you won't be willing to do all that work to keep your life going. So, that is how I keep my motivation up. I make sure to love my life. I put my goals, and dreams, and simple joys, and adventures ahead of taking care of myself, which might seem counterintuitive, but I find that if you are living for something bigger than just yourself, you end up loving your life quite a lot."

It was during her scariest experience with CF at thirteen years old that Claire's personal resolve morphed into something greater. "I went in for a routine surgery," she said, "and contracted a blood infection. Next thing I knew, my vitals were dropping, my fever was skyrocketing, and my lungs were failing in front of my eyes. There was nothing I could do. No extra treatments could fix it, and that's when I truly understood what having a terminal illness means. Having a terminal illness means that no matter how hard you work, no matter how much energy and time you put into taking care of yourself, at the end of the day, your illness will win. Of course, it didn't win this time, and I made it through a two-week coma with a one percent chance of surviving."

When Claire came to, she saw family and friends, and felt instantly grateful for the support she received. "I soon realized that other children living with CF might not have the same support that I did. That's when I decided I had to do something."

Shortly after her recovery, she founded Claire's Place Foundation, a 501(c)(3) not-for-profit organization that provides grants to enable emotional and financial support to families living with cystic fibrosis. Claire's Place Foundation has two programs: the Extended Hospital Stay Fund and the Family Support Program. For the Extended Stay Program, the foundation has set up a special cache of funds available to families with children who are experiencing a hospital stay of at least fourteen consecutive days. "Extended stays are a financial stress, and often the children are in a city far from home," said Claire.

The Family Support Program connects families living with cystic fibrosis to communicate with each other and "share their experience, strength, and hope with newly diagnosed or isolated families looking for support," said Claire. "In fact, cystic fibrosis patients cannot be in the same room with one another due to cross infection, which makes video and social media so powerful to these families."

What led to Claire starting this huge project? "When I was recovering from the coma, I was able to meet the other parents that my family had befriended in the waiting area of the PICU, who also had children on death's door," she said. "Few of the other parents had support, and struggled to manage their regular lives and other children. That was a major reason as to why I was grateful. My parents were given emotional and financial support, and were thus holding themselves together and were able to be there for me while I recovered. I felt blessed and simultaneously guilty that I had so many people looking out for my parents and little sister, while other parents who were going through the same—if not worse—situations were having to struggle just to keep their lives from falling apart.

"None of the other families were CF families, but I knew the CF world better than anything else and thought that would be a good place to start in regard to offering support. My mom took on the responsibility of caring for me 'round the clock when I was discharged from the hospital. I had three times as much medical equipment and therapies that needed doing, and she couldn't keep a stable job while caring for me, so she ended up sacrificing her career for me. While I know that 'that's just what mothers do,' and she herself would never call it a sacrifice, I think it's important to acknowledge what parents have to give up for their children when they are sick. I couldn't take the burden off my mother, but I could offer support to other mothers and fathers."

Claire remembered so many other children who affected her. "There was a little boy who used to be left alone all day and most of the night every day he was in the hospital because his parents had full-time jobs and couldn't take off two weeks of work every month or so. He stands out to me because I used to watch him make the loop around the hallways again and again and again out of boredom, and wished CF patients could hang out because I would have invited him to craft with me.

"There were patients who fought with their parents about their therapies and had no support or resources to talk out their feelings around procedures or therapies, which would oftentimes make them just shut off and refuse to take care of themselves. A lot of people don't think about the health impact of having parents that are struggling financially or emotionally. It affects us even at a young age."

While Claire oversaw her growing nonprofit, which, to date, has provided financial assistance of more than $1 million to over one hundred families, she made plenty of time for school, aspiring to study anthropology at UC Berkeley. Claire discussed a lot of her hopes in her videos, which can be found on the Claire Wineland YouTube channel.

"If you don't have CF, it is truly hard to know and understand the time I spend each day doing therapy. But, I think what those who are not living with disease with such a demanding treatment regimen don't necessarily understand is that I am so normal in so many ways. Though I am dealing with a terminal illness, I panic about tests and school, paying the bills, eating right, friends, and my future like everyone else. I spend very little time actually thinking about my illness. Healthy people always assume that my illness takes up this massive part of my life, when in reality I am over here panicking about the text message I just sent a guy I like, rather than forgetting to take pills!"

During the production of this book, Claire had a double-lung transplant. During the procedure, she had a massive stroke and went into a coma. She passed away on September 2, 2018.

Claire's mom, Melissa, says, "Claire was always too big for just me and John (Claire's dad). She was a lot of person tucked into a tiny frame."

John explains, "The thing that really hit me is that Claire seemed to embody in her life these really profound concepts, and she made it so effortless to live them. Why was she so magnetic? Why was her message so powerful? Why did she touch so many people? It wasn't just that she was sick. She took this concept of making art from your life, and she lived fully. She had this relationship with death. She made it an ally. She made every act in her life as if it was the last act on earth palpable. She used death as a way to live life fully. One of the gifts of Claire's life is that she knew that she did not have time."

We are thankful for the time she did have, because she taught us all how to live.

NATALIE WOOLF

Age at passing: 38   **Resided:** Johannesburg, Gauteng, South Africa
Age at diagnosis: A few months after birth

Natalie Woolf's legacy is unmatched in the dancing world. She won seven world championships, including three British Exhibition Championships, three World Exhibition Championships, one US Exhibition Championship, a US Millennium Championship, and two World Professional Showcase Championships. She was also the recipient of the prestigious Carl Alan Award for Performance in Theatre Arts.

"I have learned to appreciate life a lot more and embrace every tomorrow."

ELIZABETH "LIBBY" HANKINS

Age at passing: 23

Resided: Alabama, United States

Age at diagnosis: 2

Served as student council vice president, varsity cheerleader, and homecoming queen in high school; served as head cheerleader, University of West Alabama ambassador, and homecoming queen in college

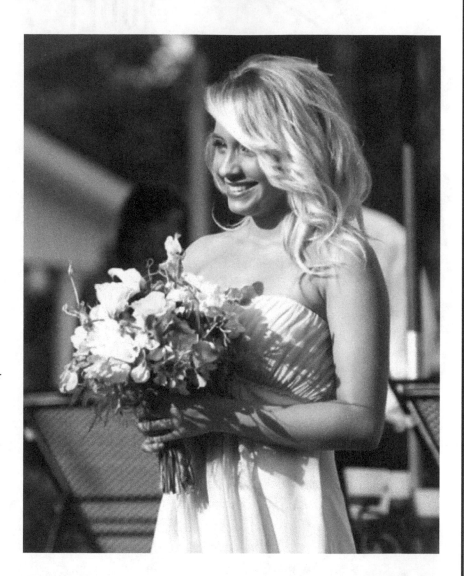

"Moments, not things, will give you strength when you need to fight, and comfort when it is time to let go."

After two years of "sick" visits to her pediatrician's office, which resulted in a "failure to thrive" diagnosis, Libby Hankins' father, Scott, took her to a local general-practice doctor, who suggested that his daughter be sweat-tested for cystic fibrosis. Libby's correct diagnosis followed shortly, and soon she and her family were on the way to Children's Hospital in Birmingham for a three-day "education" stay.

While the nurses and therapists taught Libby's family about medications, breathing treatments, and manual chest physiotherapy, Libby's mother, Susan, said the most important lesson she learned came one night when Libby's first pulmonologist and two nurse practitioners came to talk to her about life with a child with cystic fibrosis. "We had been hospitalized for two nights at this point, and I had been not only learning the basics, but also watching the other CF patients on the floor. I had noticed a difference in their attitudes. Although Libby was on a pediatric floor where everyone was relatively the same age, I noticed that some were content to be in the hospital while others talked incessantly about leaving for home, seeing their friends, or going back to school.

"When I talked to Libby's doctor about it, he told me something that I like to think shaped the course of my daughter's life. He said, 'Some of these patients are kids who have CF. Some are 'cystics.' Having CF has become the focus of their lives.' As devastating as Libby's diagnosis was, I decided at that point that my daughter would never be a 'cystic.' Having CF might mean that she would lead a 'different' life, but it would never be 'lesser.'"

Libby was typically hospitalized three times a year during elementary school, and often attended school on home IVs. She recalled her first tough time with CF, "When I was eight years old, my mom was doing my physical therapy one night and blood started running out of either corner of my mouth. I didn't know it was happening until she quickly put her hand under my chin to catch the blood. This was the first time I had ever coughed up blood. My mother immediately started packing a bag for us to go to the emergency room. She sat me in the middle hallway of our house so she could keep talking to me while she ran around nervously in all the other rooms to gather our things. She walked by, and I asked if she was scared. It stopped her in her tracks.

"She sat down beside me and asked if I was scared. I said, 'I am if you are.' She has always said that was the moment she knew that she had to be strong so that I would be able to be strong. She knew that I was learning everything about how to handle life with CF from her and how she reacted. I think she was really scared, though, because when we got to the hospital, she had packed sixteen pairs of panties for me, and she had only the ones she was wearing!"

When Libby got to high school and her disease progressed, the hospital stays grew more frequent. "We tried our best to schedule admissions around holidays," she said, "and Christmas vacation was always spent at the hospital. My doctors encouraged as much physical activity as possible, and I turned a love for gymnastics into a passion for cheerleading."

When Libby was twelve, her lung function took a rapid decline. She started IVIG therapies to strengthen her immune system, but it was obvious that something new was growing. Multiple bronchoscopies showed "untyped cepecia." While it was a scary diagnosis that upset Libby, as well as her entire family, it also made them all more vigilant and proactive about her care. Her breathing treatments and PT increased, and exercising became even more important.

"I can vividly remember cheering at football games with my home IV pump strapped to my back, because I wasn't going to miss out on a thing. I cheered all the way through high school and then went on to cheer my way through college at the University of West Alabama (UWA) in Livingston. Cheering gave me a focus and a family who has stood by me through every bump." Cheering was not easy for Libby, but she fought. Athletic trainers would pad her port before practices and games, and she would sit in class and change out IV medications.

"Libby was so strong and free. Nothing held her back, not even CF!" says Christian Morris, her old cheer partner at UWA. "She was determined and one heck of a negotiator. Hospital visits, stays, or doctor recommendations never stood a chance. She had her own terms and conditions when it came to how long she'd have to stay or if she had to stay at all. It was never about her not wanting to get better, it was all about getting back to the people and things she loved most."

Libby was able to manage a relatively "normal" life until her senior year of college. She had to withdraw to relocate to Duke University in Durham, North Carolina, to receive a double-lung transplant. She moved there in February and began daily pulmonary rehabilitation sessions and transplant classes. When she arrived at Duke, her lung function was a measly 17 percent, her temperature averaged around 103, and she was oxygen dependent. She weighed ninety-two pounds and vomited everything she put in her mouth. A feeding tube soon provided her nutrition twenty-four hours a day.

While she was waiting for her new lungs and growing weaker every day, Libby thought about all the things she had done in her life. "I remembered the big moments, like making the cheer squad for the first time, taking long car rides to clear my head, sitting in my mom's lap just to be held for a minute, holding my dogs for the first time, lying in bed having girl talks with my best friends, and singing my poor lungs out at concerts. I was clearly nearing my death, but 'things' never crossed my mind."

Scott believes her optimism was contagious. "Elizabeth was the most amazing person I have ever known, always wearing that beautiful smile and projecting positive energy, and this is what everyone fell in love with."

Susan also recalls her daughter's zest for life despite often being faced with difficult circumstances. "Libby spoke for about twenty minutes about what it is like to live with CF. Then she said, 'Now, I want you to listen carefully, because this is the most important thing I'm going to say. For every single bad thing that has ever happened to me, I can name five great ones. I get to choose how to live my life. This is my life, and I choose joy.'"

After two dry runs, Libby received her new lungs on April 17, 2016. After twelve hours in ICU, she was already breathing above the ventilator. She moved to a step-down unit in two days and was discharged to complete post-transplant therapy. After living in Durham for ten months, she returned home to Alabama in December to finish her final semester of school.

"My new lungs have given me a new life to fill with amazing adventures, but I won't ever forget what my old lungs taught me. Moments, not things, will give you strength when you need to fight, and comfort when it is time to let go."

The young Alabama native knew her standing on this earth was very finite. "When it is my time to leave this earth, I want to look back on my life and know that I lived a life full of happiness." Her mantra became "Don't count the days. Make the days count."

Libby did some pretty incredible things, but it's what she called her greatest achievement that reveals the kind of person that she was. "I believe my greatest accomplishment has come from never using CF as an excuse. I was always an A and B student and had lots of friends. When I got to high school, I became a varsity cheerleader, student council vice president, and homecoming queen. My senior year, I was awarded various scholarships for both academics and leadership. I continued cheering through college, joined Phi Mu sorority and held executive council positions, served as an orientation leader, a UWA ambassador, head cheerleader for two years, and freshman homecoming maid, and then went on to become homecoming queen. I love and am loved by the most loyal, supportive, encouraging friends and family a girl could ever have. If I stumbled, they caught me. If I grew weak in faith, they built me up. I've laughed more than I've cried. Who could ask for more than that in life?"

Libby lost her life on March 17, 2017, at Duke University Hospital, eleven months to the day of the transplant that kept her alive. In her memory, her family and friends held Kindness Week for Libby's donor, which was Libby's idea before she passed. Kindness Week is when Libby's family and friends encourage followers of the Lungs for Libby page to do random acts of kindness in honor of her donor and her donor's family. Her family and friends also formed the Live Like Libby-Love Like Libby

Foundation. In memory of Libby and her donor, the foundation supports organ-donation awareness, cystic fibrosis research, special-needs children and adults, animal rescues, and community needs. All of these things were priorities to this very special young woman.

"I want Libby's story to continue to encourage others to raise CF and organ-donor awareness and the importance of faith," says Scott. "Elizabeth Scott Hankins has always been and will always be an angel to me! We are forever grateful for her donor and their family for the gift of eleven extra months."

"Libby was truly the strongest person I've ever known," her mom remembers. "She had an incredible way of making you believe anything was possible."

HONORABLE MENTIONS

While we wish we could include every CF warrior story in this book, there is just not enough room. However, there were some people whose stories were so great that I wanted to make sure that they were acknowledged in some way. These individuals are no less CF warriors than anyone else.

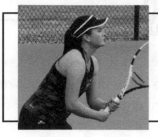

JORDAN STRICKLAND

Jordan, now a sophomore tennis player at Western Carolina University, is a four-time North Carolina state high school doubles champion.

Age: 21
Resides: North Carolina, United States
Age at diagnosis: 3 days

MATT OLIVEIRA

Age: 27
Resides: Nevada, United States
Age at diagnosis: 8 months

Matt, a flight attendant and avid adventurer, uses his social-media platform "Mystery Flights" to convey to the tens of thousands who follow him the value of dreaming big.

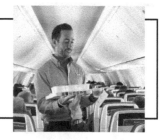

NICOLE GRAZIANO

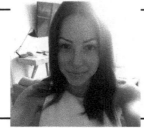

Nicole, a two-time lung-transplant recipient, owns a résumé which includes over a dozen films and a half dozen theatrical shows, including Wicked on Broadway.

Age: 29
Resides: North Carolina, United States
Age at diagnosis: 3

NATHAN CHARLES

Age: 30
Resides: Perth, Western Australia, Australia
Age at diagnosis: 3 months

Nathan has the distinction of being the first participant in a professional contact sport who has cystic fibrosis, as he played on the Australian rugby national team, the Wallabies.

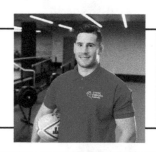

RYAN RIPLEY

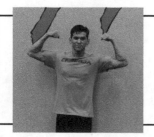

Ryan, then known as the CF Warrior and now nicknamed the CF Ninja, became the first person with cystic fibrosis to compete on the television show American Ninja Warrior.

Age: 30
Resides: Missouri, United States
Age at diagnosis: 3 months

STEVE BELL

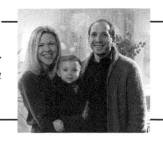

Age: 35
Resides: New Jersey, United States
Age at diagnosis: 3 months

Steve, a marathon runner and triathlete, is a member of the Ithaca College Hall of Fame for his years as a soccer standout.

ALEX PANGMAN

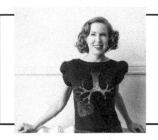

Alex, a two-time lung-transplant recipient and professional singer, was nominated for a JUNO Award (Canada's version of the Grammy Award) for an album she made just six months after her second transplant.

Age: 42
Resides: Toronto, Ontario, Canada
Age at diagnosis: Infancy

BRIAN CALLANAN

Age: 42
Resides: Florida, United States
Age at diagnosis: Birth

Brian founded the CF Lifestyle Foundation in 2003, a 501(c)(3) foundation that has provided more than one thousand CF Recreation Grants throughout the US totaling more than $500,000.

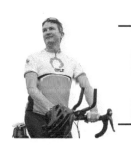

MICHAEL BURKE

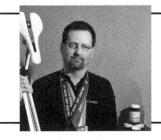

Michael, an author, running coach, and keynote speaker, has an athletic résumé that includes running an Olympic-distance triathlon, nine full marathons, and twenty half marathons.

Age: 49
Resides: Missouri, United States
Age at diagnosis: 14 months

SHELLY WEINER MAGUIRE

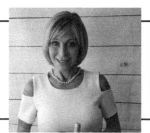

Age: 58
Resides: Florida, United States
Age at diagnosis: 12

Shelly, a motivational speaker and author, is known for being a regular presenter on the Home Shopping Network, hosting an international radio show, and developing and bringing to the market over sixty antiaging skin-care products in the past fifteen years.

EPILOGUE

After retrieving, reading, and editing hundreds of CF warriors' narratives from more than thirty countries from around the world, I picked up on some commonalities of those who have been the most successful. I call it **E.F.F.O.R.T.**

E XERCISE

Almost every single warrior considers exercise a huge part of his or her success. In this book, there are people who do some jaw-dropping things regarding exercise, but even someone who runs for just a few minutes a day seems to notice a difference!

F AITH

I'm not referring to religion, nor do most of the individuals in this book. Everyone needs to believe in something, and I've found almost every single warrior believes in him- or herself.

F AILURE

Just about every single person has dealt with bumps along the road to success. Instead of quitting, though, these champions have learned to embrace failure as a *necessity* for success.

O UTLOOK

One commonality among CF warriors that seems to stand out more than any other is a positive outlook. Our attitudes are frequently tested, but we ultimately win the battle by staying confident.

R EGIMEN

The list of medicines and therapies that each CF warrior has to follow is exhausting, yet if one is regimented, he or she stands the best chance of living a long, happy life.

T RANSPARENCY

All of the people in this book are open about sharing their stories and using those stories to help others.

AUTHOR'S FINAL NOTE

Thank you to the following people for their help with the project: Jason Serotta, Liz Buist, Peggy Davis, Priya Ramani, Jason Heaven, and Jami Kohn.

This book was written in honor of those fighters both past and present who have created hope for the next—and hopefully final—generation of cystic fibrosis warriors. Thank you for making CF stand for *can fight!*

I also want to thank all of those who bravely shared their stories, whether they were published or not. From teenagers to septuagenarians, I learned a lot on this journey. There are heroes all over this world who get little fanfare, despite the efforts they put forth. Some are fortunate to have insurance coverage, while others are fighting for just the basics to fight this disease. Some are endurance athletes, while some fight just to take a deep breath. Some are advocates who have changed the landscape of drug accessibility in their countries, while others are just trying to advocate for themselves.

They all have one thing in common: they are cystic fibrosis warriors.

We would love to hear your CF Warrior story! Connect with us on Instagram @cfwarriorproject, on Twitter @CFWarriorProj, and use the tag #cfwarrior. For more information, please visit us at CFWarriorProject.org.

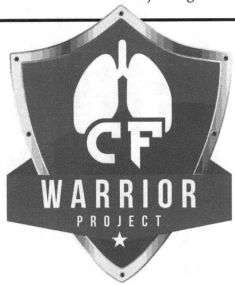

ANDY C. LIPMAN

Age: 45

Resides: Georgia, United States

Age at diagnosis: Birth

Husband; father of two; motivational speaker; author of four books; Olympic-torch bearer for the 2002 Salt Lake City Olympic Games; 2013 Turknett Leadership Award winner; 2016 Alex Award recipient; chairman of National Corporate Fundraising at the Cystic Fibrosis Foundation; emeritus board member of the Terry College at the University of Georgia; finisher of twenty-three consecutive AJC Peachtree Road Races; cofounder of the Wish for Wendy Foundation, which has raised more than $4 million to benefit the Cystic Fibrosis Foundation

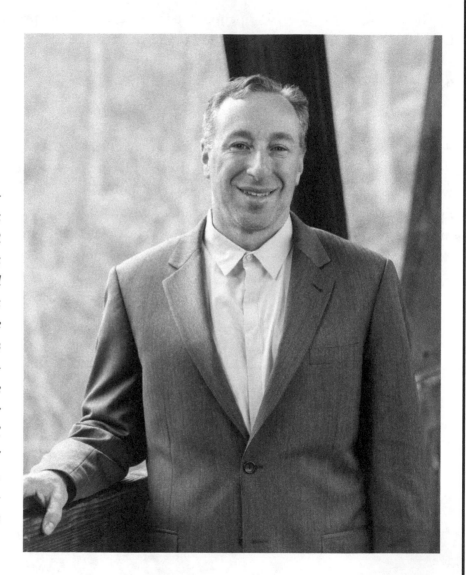

"Live your dreams and love your life."

Author Andy Lipman was born and diagnosed with cystic fibrosis in 1973, and is the author of four books primarily focused on the disease. Additionally, Lipman is a motivational speaker who goes around the world and speaks on the importance of demonstrating a positive attitude, having a sense of humor, and staying physically fit to be successful in the battle against depression, anxiety, and CF.

Lipman is a strong proponent for being compliant both with a regular exercise routine and a consistent daily medical regimen. The latter he learned from his parents, Charles and Eva, who rarely missed a day of administrating his postural drainage therapy or forcing him to take his enzymes. Lipman credits physical fitness, medical breakthroughs, and a strong support system for helping him to live to the age of forty-five, nearly triple the number he and those born during the 1970s were expected to live.

While Lipman takes pleasure in his role in the world of cystic fibrosis, he is proudest of three things: his daughter, Avery, his son, Ethan, and his wife, Andrea, who provided the inspiration for this book. He is also grateful for his younger sister, Emily, and the rest of his family and friends, who have been so supportive of his many goals.

He spends his free time rooting for his Georgia Bulldogs, Atlanta Braves, and Atlanta Falcons, coaching his children in whatever little-league sport they desire to play, and counting his lucky stars that he married the woman of his dreams.

Lipman's motto is "Live your dreams and love your life." He believes that every single warrior in this book has demonstrated those words.

THE WISH FOR WENDY FOUNDATION

Andy Lipman, along with his family and friends, created the Wish for Wendy Softball Challenge in October of 2000 in memory of his older sister, Wendy Carol Lipman, who passed away from cystic fibrosis in 1971 after living only sixteen days.

Due to the success of the tournament, Lipman and his family founded the Wish for Wendy Foundation in August of 2006, a nonprofit organization dedicated to increasing awareness about living with cystic fibrosis and supporting efforts to find a cure. Like the Wish for Wendy Softball Challenge, the foundation is in memory of Lipman's older sister, Wendy. In nineteen years, the Wish for Wendy Foundation and the softball tournament have raised more than $4 million to benefit the Cystic Fibrosis Foundation, making the latter one of the largest charity softball tournaments in the United States.

Our wish for Wendy is that one day people with cystic fibrosis will no longer have to struggle with this disease.

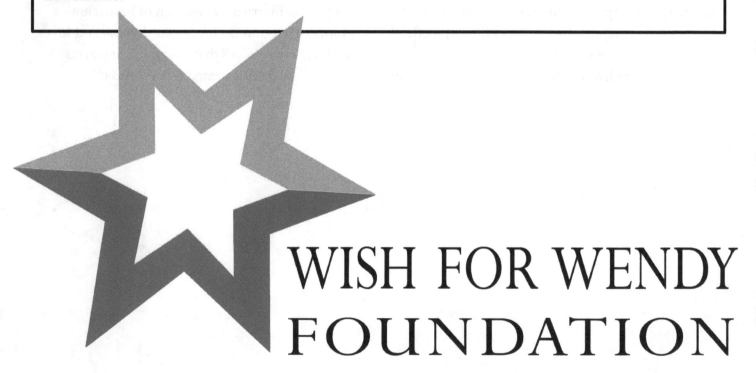

WISH FOR WENDY
FOUNDATION